Small Remedies &
Interesting Cases II

PROCEEDINGS OF THE 1990 PROFESSIONAL CASE CONFERENCE

Editors: Stephen King, ND, DHANP
Sheryl Kipnis, ND, DHANP
Cathie Scott

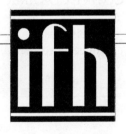

International
Foundation
for
Homeopathy

INTERNATIONAL FOUNDATION FOR HOMEOPATHY

The IFH is a nonprofit organization dedicated to promoting the public awareness of classical homeopathy and to maintaining the highest standards of homeopathic practice and education by means of public and professional courses, research, and working toward the establishment of homeopathic medical schools.

OFFICE

2366 Eastlake Avenue E., Suite 301, Seattle, WA 98102 • (206) 324-8230

BOARD OF DIRECTORS

OFFICERS

EXECUTIVE CO-DIRECTORS

Copyright © 1990 by The International Foundation for Homeopathy

ISBN 0-8403-6636-1

Printed in the United States of America
10 9 8 7 6 5 4 3 2 1

WITH GRATEFUL THANKS

A portion of the editorial and printing costs of this publication was underwritten by generous grants from the following organizations:

- Charles M. Bauervic Foundation

- Boiron-Borneman

- Standard Homeopathic Company

On behalf of all homeopathic practitioners and patients, and for all others who will benefit from the information preserved here, the IFH would like to thank these organizations for their kind assistance.

ACKNOWLEDGEMENTS

We extend thanks to Dean Crothers, MD, for his help in preparing some of the computerized case analyses for publication; Anne Walton Design and Lillian Sugahara, for the graphic design and typesetting; and Mariel Damaskin, of Kendall/Hunt Publishing, for general assistance.

In particular, Drs. King and Kipnis would like to thank co-editor Cathie Scott for many long hours of editorial work in helping to make this book a reality.

And, most of all, thanks to each conference speaker for sharing so instructively from your clinical experience. Each prescriber polishes a unique facet of the gem that is homeopathy, and that gem shines brighter because of your individual contribution.

TABLE OF CONTENTS

PREFACE

It is one thing to do something well the first time. It is quite another to do it successfully again. And so, it is with considerable satisfaction and a sense of real accomplishment that all of us here at the International Foundation for Homeopathy bring this second book of cured cases to the community of homeopathic prescribers and enthusiasts around the world.

The 1990 IFH Professional Case Conference, held in Seattle in early June, was a worthy successor to our first conference in 1989. There was plenty of excitement among both the presenting speakers and their audience of homeopathic colleagues. The clinical information generated by the conference was at a consistently high level, and the discussions were stimulating indeed.

In publishing this material, our goal is once again simple: we want to preserve this valuable information for all present and future homeopaths.

Plans are already in motion for the 1991 conference. We intend to continue publishing each year's proceedings so that the passage of time will bring a growing list of volumes, each one making another contribution to the common body of homeopathic knowledge.

Perhaps a word about the notations used in the cases would be helpful for some readers. While taking cases, homeopaths often underline symptoms for emphasis. A given symptom may be underlined zero, one, two, or three times, depending on the intensity, clarity, and spontaneity of the symptom as given by the patient. The strongest emphasis is represented by a symptom underlined three times.

In this book the underlining is given as a number in parentheses after the symptom. Thus, "irritable in the morning on waking (3)" means that the homeopath felt this was a strong symptom in the patient's case, and it was therefore underlined three times for emphasis. If no number follows a particular symptom, then the symptom was not underlined by the homeopath.

Stephen King, ND, DHANP
Sheryl Kipnis, ND, DHANP

Murray Feldman, MCH, RS Hom

A CASE OF RAYNAUD'S PHENOMENON
AND
A CASE OF DEPRESSION

Murray Feldman, MCH, RS Hom, is a graduate of the College of Homeopathy, London, England, and a registered member of the Society of Homeopaths, United Kingdom. Murray has been studying, practicing, and teaching homeopathy in India and England since 1977. He is now practicing and teaching homeopathy in Vancouver, British Columbia, Canada.

Introduction

I was talking with a friend and homeopathic colleague recently about the fact that both of us like detective and suspense movies. We felt that we could not resist liking them because we are like detectives, always looking for clues as to what is characteristic in our patients. So, when I was asked for a title for Case Number 1, I inwardly resisted defining it with a clinical label and would have preferred some detective-style name such as "The Case of the Held-Back Heart with the Cold Hands." To me, this title captures the dynamic nature of the case. And, after all, we treat and cure living people, not static diseases.

As homeopaths, we are very fortunate to be able to look at the deeper aspects of people, to see clinical results for what they are; to see cases from first to last, from the inner to the outer; and to be able to truly focus on the dynamic process of the patient before us. Our philosophy and methodology both allow and require us to do this.

I believe it is important to remember that we really do not know all that much about either homeopathy or the patient. Because of this, I am always looking for new ways to more accurately perceive the patient. One way that has been useful to me in grasping the essence of a case is based on the approach described by Joseph Reves, an Israeli homeopath. I heard about it from some of his students in France.

Reves emphasizes the idea of "simple language." Through the words that patients use to tell their stories, something characteristic about each person (and the remedy required) is revealed.

For example, here are some statements from a case I took recently:

"I have a friend recently diagnosed with cancer. I think she's going to cash it in soon."

"I've been doing some work on myself and it's starting to pay dividends."

"Whenever I get angry, I see that I have to buy back that anger from my childhood."

Just from this man's language we know something about him — about his priorities, about his fears.

Here is another example from a case I took in England recently: "Whenever I am criticized, it's like a knife cutting me up.... One part of me is in Denmark with my family, and the other part of me is over here in England." The words are so indicative of this person's subjective state. He repeatedly used words referring to cutting and dividing.

Language is very important to us in homeopathy. Patients express themselves in words and images which can lead us to correct understanding and, thus, to correct prescriptions. I'd like you to keep this in mind as we look at the two cases I am presenting today. Both are very rich in words and images.

Case Number 1: A Case of Raynaud's Phenomenon

Miss R.
Single
Born: March 13, 1963

Initial Visit: June 1986

My hands get very cold; they can ache as if the blood is cut off (3). They freeze in the winter. They seem to get cold when I feel I have a lot to say in my heart.

My sinuses get blocked; they seem to swell up.

My period has gotten a bit more uncomfortable lately, a much heavier flow (2) the last five months. A 28-day cycle with a five-day flow.

I got bad sinuses when I visited my mother last. She (my mother) lived her life off of her children, with a fear of losing them. She was closest with me when younger. I liked that role. When I was very young, she wasn't around; until I was eight, she was very busy. My father died when I was 11. The others left home. Suddenly, there was just me and my mom. She's encouraging of me, but makes statements like "All judgment is suspended. I've got you in hold."

My brother drowned at age six.

I didn't know how to be a child. I learned to be calm; underneath I was frustrated. Could never express myself as a child. There was never room for me to say anything in the house, so I would do things to get attention, like trying to please my family. I used to wear funny clothes, the freak of the family.

The blocked snuffly nose started when I was six or seven years old. My nose gets totally plugged, but nothing ever comes out (2).

Cold hands ever since I can remember. My hands get numb, cold, as if they will drop off (2). Worse during the winter. They ache when I feel connected with inner love and can even feel warm inside. I hate the winter (3).

I can be clumsy, knocking things over, not spatially aware. My hands don't work well. I get jumbled between left and right hands. I always had to balance things out: one toe, the other toe (2). This incoordination thing is a big deal (3). I used to do juggling and balancing to overcome it.

My hands can go purple and blue and white at times. I can't go under the water for a long time without my ears aching.

History of chicken pox, mumps, swollen submaxillary glands.

My words don't always flow easily. As a child, I used to stutter. It can still happen. It is difficult to get words off my tongue. I come from a very intellectual family; what one said was important. If we sat at the table with the big ones, we had to be quiet. There was a lot of emphasis on being articulate or shutting up. I was a chatterbox when I was younger. I would find group discussions excruciating. My whole self-worth was based on what I could contribute in the group. I would feel safest if I could control. I had to feel I was indispensable and had a definite role, or I'd be left out.

My memory of my father is as a statue. He was an invalid for the last five years of his life. He was a politician before that, not home a lot. We were made to feel we were lucky to be with dad. We had to look up to him. He would only appreciate you when you could look up to him in an intelligent manner. If you don't behave, you're lucky to be with him. I felt walked out on by him at times.

I'm always the one who is wrong. I take the blame on myself. I am distrustful of pointing things out; I would assume it was my fault.

Anger when I feel my older brother isn't listening to me.

I went to boarding school for high school. I have fears that I'm a big creep and everyone hates me and I'll be totally isolated (2).

As a child, when we had to sit at separate tables to eat, I felt isolated, neglected, out in the cold.

I have a fear of the sea; it's so dark and powerful.

I have found sex fearful; fear of being overwhelmed. Also, a feeling I had to do it.

When I was swimming recently, people commented that I do it the hardest way possible. Like when throwing a ball, I push it instead of throwing it.

Going to boarding school made me feel special; I'd be treated well when I came home.

Desires sweets (1) and sour.

I have images at times of being driven or hounded across ice.

Analysis of Case Number 1

After taking Case Number 1, I really didn't have a clue as to what to prescribe. What struck me about the patient, however, was the coldness, the awkwardness, and the contraction or "held-backness." I felt they were all related. The awkwardness stood up as a general aspect of the case, indicated by the following statements, as well as other phrases:

"I didn't know how to be a child...could never express myself as a child."

"I can be clumsy, knocking things over, ..."

"This incoordination thing is a big deal."

"My words don't always flow easily. As a child I used to stutter."

"With the ball, I push it instead of throwing it."

The coldness, of course, runs throughout the case: the lack of vital heat, cold hands, hates the winter, and worse during the winter.

In repertorizing this case, the first two rubrics I used were EXTREMITIES, awkwardness, and GENERALITIES, lack of vital heat. The next rubric was the chief complaint, EXTREMITIES, icy cold hands. I also used the rubric, NOSE, coryza, without a discharge. I thought this was a good particular symptom that also reflected the essential contracted nature of the case. She was fearful of sex and recently had an increased, heavy menstrual flow, so I added this recent change, FEMALE GENITALIA, copious menses. On repertorization of these five rubrics, the following remedies came through in all of them: Nux vomica, Causticum, Camphor, Arsenicum album, Agaricus, Lachesis, and Natrum carbonicum.

I wanted, if possible, to eliminate some of these remedies from consideration. Looking again at the case, I saw a large element of isolation, which was related very much to the state of contraction and coldness:

"My memory of my father is as a statue." (What a powerful feeling this image conjures up in relation to the rest of the case.)

"I felt walked out on by him at times."

"As a child, we had to sit at separate tables to eat. I felt isolated, neglected, out in the cold. I have fears...that I'll be totally isolated."

I added another rubric, MIND, forsaken. I wasn't sure if this was a valid rubric, but I used it with a kind of curiosity. The following three remedies came through all six symptoms: Camphor, Lachesis, and Natrum carbonicum. I could see nothing to confirm Lachesis and Natrum carbonicum, but Camphor was an interesting possibility.

When I think of Camphor, I think first of coldness. The case itself was also filled with coldness. The patient's own words, phrases such as "being driven or hounded across ice," provided powerful images of coldness.

Coldness, isolation, and contraction or cramping are essential features of Camphor and were very profound in this case. I also discovered the symptom "Awkwardness" listed for Camphor in the GENERALITIES section of Phatak's materia medica.

Plan: I decided to give Camphor 200c.

Results of Camphor Prescription in Case Number 1

First Follow-Up: October 29, 1986

Incredibly, I don't feel that strangling feeling in my hands anymore.

Energy changed after the remedy.

I used to be so clumsy; I don't feel that way anymore. After the remedy, I felt very clumsy for one week. I then forgot about being clumsy; just remembered that I used to be that way.

I have become more playful, and have more sexual energy.

Still blocked in sinuses.

Feel more grounded.

No one comments on my cold hands anymore.

The coordination thing isn't an issue anymore.

Still feel afraid of sex, but feeling more comfortable with my femininity. Wearing clothes that fit me now, rather than baggy and hiding.

Feel less fearful of putting self forward. Last two menses more painful, but regular.

Joints crack less.

Plan: Wait. No remedy given.

Second Follow-Up: November 2, 1986

Some return of cold hand symptoms.

Plan: Repeat Camphor 200c.

Third Follow-Up: December 17, 1986

No problems at all with coldness.

Feeling more weepy, open.

Sinuses a little better.

Periods normal.

I'm starting to see how much I put myself down.

Plan: Wait. No remedy given.

(This woman has had no return of the original complaint since this time and has felt no need to have another remedy. She has done very well indeed. It is interesting to note that the cracking of the joints, which she reported as better in the first follow-up, wasn't brought out in the initial case. Yet the repertory lists Camphor in italics for this symptom, further confirming the prescription.)

Case Number 2: A Case of Depression

Miss S.
Single
Born: March 20, 1960

Initial Visit: December 1987

Depressed; very tired all the time (3). My sleep is extremely restless but I don't feel like getting up and facing the day.

I feel lonely, cut off and numb (2). I don't even feel like communicating with people. I feel very alienated and alone, as if there is no one out there for me. At times it's as if there is no one else left at all (2). I had a three-year relationship that ended recently and also lost my job. I think I've always been like this to some degree or other, but never so bad. Even in school I was a loner pretty much. I don't remember my parents being there for me. My memories of them are cold and absent. The world seems like a cold, barren place to me (3).

It's strange. I never thought about religion much, but lately I've been thinking about God. I wonder if I should pray, but I don't think that would even help me. I feel abandoned by God, and I feel there is no hope for me, no way out (3).

I'd like to have someone to talk to, but I don't really think they'd care for me that much. I keep wondering what I can do to get out of this. Can you help me? I find when friends do talk to me to try to help, I just seem to argue. I can't help myself. I don't get that angry; I just don't agree with them and the suggestions they make. We seem to have opposite viewpoints (1).

Losing my boyfriend was a real blow. I thought we might marry. He just seemed to lose interest. I have no real interests. I worked for an insurance agency, as a secretary. They said they couldn't afford to keep me.

Desires sweets (3) and spice.

Averse to fats (1).

I feel the cold a lot and really need to dress warm (2). Cold hands and feet, but at times I can feel warm inside. And hands and feet feel cold to touch, not to me, but I hate the cold.

I want to stay indoors and rest. When I think about how I am and that I should do something, I freeze. I can't find anything to do to help save me.

Tends toward sluggish bowels. For the last three to four months has had cramps in the stomach (pointed to her abdomen), especially before bowel motions (1).

Menses are regular, lasting for five days and occurring every 28 days. They have never been a problem.

Used to have strong sexual desire, but lately this has decreased to nothing.

Plan: Pulsatilla 1M.

First Follow-Up: January 1988

No better.

Feels depressed and tired.

Hopeless.

Low energy.

Analysis of Case Number 2

My first remedy in this case, without use of the repertory, was Pulsatilla, based on the "sinned away her day of grace" idea, the aversion to fats, the loneliness, and an element of manipulative self-pity. It was obvious, however, on looking over the case again, especially the weather modalities, that Pulsatilla didn't sufficiently cover the entire case. My second choice initially was Aurum metallicum. With the failure of Pulsatilla, I decided to study the case, to carefully select rubrics, and to repertorize, rather than just prescribing Aurum.

This case is also rich in language expressing the central theme of coldness, loneliness, and "held-backness." I felt the most important two rubrics were MIND, forsaken ("I feel lonely, cut-off, numb, alienated, alone, as if there is no one there for me.") and MIND, despair of religious salvation. This despair was something she had never thought about, but now it was extremely marked: "I feel abandoned by God, no hope for me, no way out." I also used the rubric, MIND, contrary, because she doesn't agree with her friends: "We seem to have opposite viewpoints." Other rubrics that portray this contracted state are GENERALITIES, lack of vital heat; ABDOMEN, cramping; and FEMALE GENITALIA, diminished sex drive.

Camphor was the only remedy that came through the six rubrics. Lachesis, Aurum, and Argentum nitricum were next. Of these three, Aurum was the only one I considered. It's interesting that Lachesis came high on repertorization in both cases, but I don't know what it means.

There is much that can be said for giving Aurum in this case: the history of grief, the long periods of loneliness and depression, religious despair, loss of job, and cold feet and hands. Who knows what it would have done?

I did, however, look up Camphor in Allen's encyclopedia and found the following:

Desire to dispute, self-willed.

I was alone in the great universe, the last of all things, there was no other feeling in my soul than that of my hopeless endless damnation. I sank back upon the bed, believing that I was the spirit of evil in a world forsaken by God. Faith and hope were gone. My misery was boundless...hopelessly devoted to everlasting damnation...I cried out aloud, "And so I am dead, that hell I used to think about is no fiction." And yet I confessed this very morning and no heavy sin rests upon my conscience.... the time seemed an eternity and the most painful thought was that I was forever deprived of Divine protection and of every consolation and every hope. Nothing remained to me but the conviction of my everlasting damnation.

This description in Allen shows a belief that the prover feels that he is evil, which my patient did not feel. But the description of isolation and eternal damnation and the coldness, along with a small rubric, MIND, delusion, alone in the world, led me to give Camphor.

Plan: Camphor 1M.

By the way, I read a case recently where Hura braziliensis was given with this sense of loneliness as the leading indication.

Results of the Camphor Prescription in Case Number 2

Case Number 2 was a very exciting and interesting case. Unfortunately, I did not get the opportunity for follow-up over a long period. Nevertheless, I feel that the clear benefit evidenced in the first follow-up after the Camphor was given illustrates that there was a curative reaction to the remedy.

March 1988

Feeling much better.

Energy increased greatly.

I can look at my friends now and talk to them. I don't feel so lost and alone anymore.

Cramping during my period, which I've never had before. Abdominal cramps are still there, but not a real problem.

I still get periods of loneliness and depression, but I'm generally feeling much less cut off and more friendly.

Still very chilly.

Plan: Wait

Summary

My knowledge of Camphor before these two cases was basically as an acute remedy, where coldness, cramps, convulsions, weakness, collapse, and mental anguish are prominent. As we all know, it was one of Hahnemann's three major remedies in treating cholera or cholera-like conditions. Its use is well-known for the beginning of colds or for feverish conditions that exhibit extreme chilliness, usually associated with restlessness.

These are my only two chronic cases of Camphor, so I am not going to make any pronouncements on Camphor or create an essence out of them. However, there are some common features that we can clearly see: the history of isolation and "cut-offness"; the contracted state; a language rich in images describing the coldness, numbness, constriction, aloneness, and alienation; and a closing down on some level.

Both cases also have unusual temperature elements to them. Case Number 1 had at times a warm heart, which of course was a feeling of love, but those were her words. The warm heart was accompanied by cold hands and feeling warm inside, yet averse to cold. Case Number 2 also mentioned that, in spite of being a chilly person, at times she had cold extremities, could feel warm inside, but hated the cold. In the provings, Camphor also has an unusual temperature element. They can be very cold to the touch with an aversion to covers and, at the same time that they are cold, can have internal burning heat. I actually was not aware of this common element in the cases and how it related to the provings until I prepared for this conference.

Jessica Jackson: In the Chinese pharmacopoeia, Camphor is said to open the orifices of the heart.

Feldman: Oh, that's very appropriate in relation to these cases. That's very nice. Thank you.

It would be interesting to hear if anyone else has had any successful Camphor cases. It seems to be a remedy that goes into the deeper, darker, primal fears of humankind: the fears associated with aloneness, despair, unworthiness, and coldness — along with feelings of separation from the world, from friends, and from the Divine.

Jennifer Jacobs: Your description of the Camphor mental state — the isolation and constriction — makes me think of patients with arthritis. The mental picture is often similar. And Camphor does have rheumatic symptoms. Boericke mentions rheumatic pain between the shoulders, cracking in the joints, and difficult motion. Perhaps we ought to think of this remedy more often for our arthritic patients.

Feldman: An interesting idea. Has anyone else had a chronic case of Camphor? The only other case I've encountered is one that Roger Morrison treated, a chronic cystitis case, I believe. It's interesting to note that Camphor and Cantharis are listed as complementary remedies.

Jo Daly: I've had one Camphor case, a patient with mental symptoms similar to those in your second case. One of the symptoms that led me to choose Camphor was that she said she felt very cold on the outside, yet she was wearing a summer dress and it was winter in England when I took the case. This is very characteristic. She did not want to cover herself up, even though she felt very chilly.

Feldman: Thank you very much.

Louis Klein, RS Hom

THREE CASES OF POST-INFLUENZAL CHRONIC FATIGUE SYNDROME

Louis Klein, RS Hom, has been studying and practicing homeopathy since 1978. He is an auxiliary teacher in the IFH Professional Course and in the Hahnemann College of Homeopathy course. Lou is a registered member of the Society of Homeopaths, United Kingdom. He has studied with George Vithoulkas and currently practices and teaches homeopathy in Vancouver, British Columbia, Canada.

Introductory Remarks

Chronic Fatigue Syndrome, Epstein-Barr, or Myalgic Encephalomyelitis are terms that refer to the relatively pervasive phenomenon of post-viral syndromes. To allopaths, the existence and extent of this phenomenon seem absolutely new. Even though these syndromes are now recognized diagnoses, controversy still exists over their credibility. Many allopaths relegate the diagnosis to a nebulous realm of non-pathological conditions that suggest hypochondriasis. In my experience, it is not unusual to see patients with these syndromes given tranquilizers and psychotropic drugs, with the idea that they are psychiatric problems.

To homeopaths, the extent to which this phenomenon has grown is not surprising. Also not surprising is the difficulty that allopaths are having in recognizing general limiting symptoms, such as fatigue and weakness, as important pathological entities. General symptoms are something homeopaths can cure, and therefore they have always had a prominent place in our repertories, materia medicas, and case management. We don't necessarily have to wait until a pathology appears and is diagnosed in order to take effective action. Also, we know that this realm of general limitation can be as serious as any pathological condition. We even take hypochondriasis seriously. We do not denigrate it as something imaginary or as some static, immovable psychiatric entity with all the conventional stigmas.

The present growth of post-viral syndromes and chronic fatigue, resulting from a weakening of the immune system, is not surprising, considering what is currently put into the human body in the name of medicine. I believe we are now seeing the results of the destructive and continuous allopathic drugging of our generation. It has been only our generation, the so-called yuppie generation, that has been exposed to so much modern medication, especially antibiotics. This relatively unlimited use of drugs resulted from our wealth, the availability of drugs, and a kind of misdirected concern that sought to treat every condition with the latest wonder drug.

Although some of these allopathic drugs have prevented mortality that could have resulted from serious infections, they have also created a sharp rise in the level of morbidity or chronic disease. The "in moderation" boundaries in which our modern, over-consumptive society and profit-driven pharmaceutical companies were operating in the past have gradually shifted. It is common now to hear that someone has taken antibiotics for minor problems such as recurrent colds and minor skin eruptions.

As homeopaths, we see conditions, pathological or not, as part of a life-long continuum of positive/nurturing or negative/destructive influences on the vital force. If simple infections are treated with antibiotics, the natural process that eliminates disease is aborted. Eventually, the body's own ability to create homeostasis is deeply affected, and the vital force's ability to maintain itself is diminished. A chronic "fatigue" results, in conjunction with other types of stresses.

Even before the introduction of antibiotics and other modern infection abortives, homeopaths recognized that a chronic sequela can result from influenza in a susceptible person. We have many references to this in our older materia medicas and repertories. This specific homeopathic information can be used as part of our strategy for treating patients with a chronic sequela.

Disease symptoms are part of a larger continuum, and any polycrest remedy can be used for post-influenzal syndromes. However, to prescribe correctly, it is important to determine if the influenza, as a causative factor, is in fact the most important and primary component of the case under consideration. In other words, the homeopath must determine if the flu (or any acute process) has grafted a new remedy imprint onto the individual, or if the symptoms and fatigue following the influenza continue to be in the curative realm of the remedy the individual may have needed prior to the influenza.

Recently, I saw two patients in the same week on follow-up. Their chief complaint was chronic fatigue syndrome, a serious weakness with other symptoms following the flu. Both patients had a remarkable, dramatic improvement of their symptoms following the administration of Stramonium. Now, this remedy is not much known for chronic fatigue syndrome, or even for fatigue or weakness alone. But the history and totality of the symptomatology led me to prescribe this remedy.

By the way, both patients complained of severe weakness starting at noon each day, a modality that Stramonium is listed under in the generalities section of Kent's repertory. Also, both had a more involved story to tell, which fell under the curative powers of Stramonium.

I would say that, along with Curare, Stramonium is an important post-viral remedy, especially where there is a history of abuse, fear, or violent anger. Also, it is my experience that the idea of prolonged abuse, fear, and violence in the past (sometimes distant) is a strong component of many cases of post-viral myelitis in general. Other contributing factors include any activities that are excessive, continuous, and depleting such as workaholism and excessive physical training.

In the Stramonium cases I have mentioned, there were Stramonium-type symptoms prior to the acute process, and these continued after the patients developed acute flus and their sequelae. The homeopath's job is to take the case as thoroughly as possible and to understand the full extent of the problem. Whether it's a Stramonium case, a Sulphur case, a Pulsatilla case, or another of our many remedies, this deeper search reveals a larger story, a "picture" of a remedy. This remedy then may be termed by some as "constitutional."

However, we may also run into the situation where we have very little information to prescribe on, except that, in the case of a "chronic fatigue syndrome," the patient truly has simply suffered a chronic weakness and a set of symptoms following the flu. In these types of cases, the flu then becomes the important factor in our case analysis.

In the following cases, ask yourself which of these case analysis strategies will give us our curative remedy.

Case Number 1

Female
Age 47
Homemaker and Part-Time Salesperson

Initial Visit

The patient reported recurrent sore throats and colds, which she terms the flu (3). It all started 15 years ago after a severe flu; then, each year from May to October she "gets a flu virus." With this flu, she gets hot and uptight, with a general feeling of sickness. This flu especially settles in the face. She gets a fullness, a weighted feeling in her face and forehead; she feels off balance; and she has a ringing in her ears (2), which can keep her awake. In the past, her visual focus was poor on turning the head. Her head gets cold in the wind, and her ears ring (2).

She is anxious before doing things (3). When she does them, it's okay. The anxiety is especially associated with the flu.

Prior to the flu, 15 years ago, her tonsils were removed because of recurring tonsillitis and sinusitis. Had taken antibiotics, decongestants, tranquilizers, and other medications for these symptoms.

Has a part-time job, 1 1/2 days per week.

Doesn't drink or smoke; good lifestyle.

Others see her as very cool, but inside she is upset and very uptight, especially in the past. This feeling is accompanied by heart palpitations and anxiety. Has never told anyone, not even her husband, about this anxiety. With a cold or flu, the anxiety (3) comes on. Then she feels she can't do things. "I can't do this or that. I don't relax."

She is always worrying (3) about something else, especially in the future. Suddenly gets worried that she can't function or gets the feeling she can't function and that the other person will notice this.

Still fears going out for dinner or even to a shopping mall. "I can't relax and be content." Always thinking ahead. Worries and goes through future scenarios (3).

Spent 20 years as a homemaker; it's a menial job. Makes all the household decisions; husband doesn't participate. Feels somewhat confident in herself because husband expects her to do this, but not as confident as others think she is. Did a lot of volunteer work. Didn't just stay at home.

Worries that she doesn't feel well and is going to get sick. The anxiety started when she had all these flus.

She has two children, who are normal. Broke her coccyx with the birth of her son. One miscarriage, at three months.

Is very organized and plans ahead. Fastidious (2).

Her problems started four or five years after her children were born; had too many commitments, even though she didn't feel well.

Fears being in airplanes (2), public speaking (3), crowds (2), being trapped in small places (2), and shopping malls (1). Feels better when she is occupied (2).

Worse from heat and sun; gets lightheaded (2). Too hot on exertion (2). Warm-blooded (1); gets flushes of heat. Sensitive to air conditioning (1).

She is sleepless from worry; can't get to sleep (2). Wakes tired (2).

Even if sick, she does all her duties. Feels appreciated by her family.

Three years prior to her problems starting, her father died unexpectedly. Then she worried about her mother, who died three years ago. The responsibility for her mother became a big stress; had lots of guilt. She is hard on herself (2).

Abdominal gas (2). Stomach aches two hours after eating; worse with raw vegetables (2).

Avoids sweets and "bad" foods (2).

Regular menses.

Good memory.

For the last three months, since March, she has had the "flu," with sore throats, stomach problems (nausea), dizziness, and a feeling of being off balance (2).

Sleeps on her left or right side.

Averse to loud music (1).

Doesn't express herself to others.

Her nervousness creates frequent urination.

Her feet perspire (1).

Doesn't cry a lot; works things out in her mind.

Does things even though she's not feeling well.

Has stomach problems, which are better with heat and worse 10 to 11 p.m.

When she has the flu, she drools; salivated with last flu; salivates after drinking fluids (2).

No energy with heat and worse from the sun (2).

During the flu, she is sensitive to both extremes of temperature.

Could talk to her mother about a problem; husband isn't sympathetic enough.

When not feeling well, she feels pressure from not getting things accomplished and the narrow range of what she can accomplish.

Family History:
- Mother: aneurysm and heart problems.
- Father: heart problems.
- Maternal Grandmother: died of cancer at age 90.
- Maternal Grandfather: died at age 40; cause is unknown.
- Paternal Grandmother: died of old age; was generally healthy.
- Paternal Grandfather: died at age 50-60; cause is unknown.

Impression: The patient was pleasant, but it was hard to confirm her symptoms and to get modalities. She was rather confused and rambling (jumped back to other symptoms). She had a friendly skepticism about homeopathy and asked a lot of questions.

Analysis of Case Number 1

This is a difficult case. Why? Because, in my mind, when I hear that someone is suffering from a post-viral problem 15 years after having the initial influenza attack, it diminishes the emphasis or value of that causative symptom. I take what the patient says seriously. But I also know that, especially in North America, a diagnosis (even a self-diagnosis) is like a sacred blessing that patients feel has been bestowed upon them, and they may cherish this as a way to ignore the deeper causes of their illness.

On the other hand, the word "flu" is repeated in this recorded case 11 times! This makes it harder to ignore. In this instance, I chose not to ignore it. I assessed that this was one of those cases where the persistent imprint of the flu was an acceptable and necessary component of the remedy I would choose.

Another important consideration, especially when one decides to choose a remedy that is not a common polycrest, is what is not in the case. When you feel uncomfortable choosing any polycrest, then search for something else! A simple idea, but many of us tend to choose that which is more comfortable and then try to fit a square peg into a round hole, with mediocre results. (More on these mediocre results later.) So, what is not in the case is as important as what is in the case. What is not in this case gives us very little with which to confirm a polycrest prescription.

The general major or primary limiting factors in this woman's life are as follows:

- Recurrent sore throats, colds, and flus.
- Anxiety.
- Sleeplessness.
- Gas.
- Being "off balance," a dizziness, with nausea.

Now, when looking at the case in order to prescribe a remedy, other symptoms and modalities come up. These symptoms and modalities make it difficult to confirm common or polycrest remedies through repertorization. So, I chose a remedy based on materia medica knowledge—knowledge not contained in the repertory. Searching remedies following the flu, I found Scutellaria lateriflora, commonly called skullcap.

The following are some of the more important symptoms I chose from a description of this remedy in Boericke's materia medica:

- "This is a nervous sedative, where nervous fear predominates."
- "Nervous weakness after the flu."
- "Fear of some calamity."
- "Inability to fix attention."
- "Confusion."
- "Dull frontal headache."
- "Restless sleep and frightful dreams."
- "Nausea."
- "Gas, fullness and distention."
- "Night terrors, sleeplessness."

Plan: Scutellaria lateriflora 200c, one dose.

Long-Term Follow-Up on Case Number 1

This woman had a dramatic improvement in all her symptoms, including her mental and emotional state and her general energy. Approximately one year later, she started having recurrent and specific sinus infections (without a recurrence of any of her mental and emotional symptoms), which were then treated with Dulcamara. She has been fine now for the past five years.

Audience: Why was Dulcamara given?

Klein: I do not have the detailed notes here, but there were specific symptoms. The pathology was just in the sinuses, and it was affected by cold and wet. There were a few other modalities of Dulcamara. Even in this original case, there is an element of Dulcamara. She had a lot of anxiety about her family.

Audience: In coming up with the remedy for a particular patient, do you feel that the etiology of a previous bout with influenza is important?

Klein: In some cases it is, and in other cases it isn't. It may be the only component that you can use in analyzing the case. And, of course, I am talking about case analysis. I am not talking about how the pathology developed, because we see symptoms and pathology as a continuum. But, in terms of analyzing a case, it is sometimes very important to identify a causative factor. Often patients may have needed Stramonium one year ago, but they go along and get this terrible flu, for which they might have needed Bryonia. They get over the flu but they still need Stramonium, even though now they are complaining about weakness, which they did not have prior to the flu.

Audience: I guess I'm still just a little confused. If what we are trying to do is match a symptom picture as it is presented to us by a patient and come up with the appropriate remedy, then what difference does it make if we think cognitively about what the predisposing or causative factor was? For instance, in this case, the bout with a viral influenza doesn't seem to matter nearly as much as the actual symptoms that the patient is presenting with in your office. You could have six people who have contracted an influenza virus and who all present with different symptom pictures, and each will require a different remedy. So what is the significance?

Klein: The significance is that homeopathy is very young. Our information about some of our medicines is rather sketchy. I wish we had a picture of each of our remedies so broad that we would have no need to inquire about past causalities. Sometimes we are like detectives. We use any little clue that we can come up with. Ultimately, we may use a particular clue, but we have to match it with the set of symptoms that is there. At this stage in our development and the development of the materia medica, we simply do not have all the information about all the remedies.

So, when I see a small note in Boericke that says, "nervous weakness after influenza," it sticks in my mind. Maybe this remedy will be useful for someone that has had influenza. We don't know that much about Scutellaria. You see? It is a tiny bit of information, but it is an important piece of information at the moment. Our materia medica has not even approached its full and true potential. It remains for us and those who come after to accomplish this.

That was a good question. Thank you.

Case Number 2

Male
Age 36
English Teacher

Initial Visit

The patient was healthy until age 32. He was a competitive runner and athlete. Eleven years ago, he noticed that he would get more flus and congestion during the winter. These flus or colds were usually preceded by an intense physical session or getting wet and chilled by jogging in bad weather. He would be worse after sweating in cold weather.

Two years ago, he got severely ill with flu-like symptoms after a hard run. He never got better and was diagnosed with Epstein-Barr and Chronic Fatigue Syndrome.

Current symptoms:

Fatigue (3).

He has dizziness (2), which is worse on awakening (2); has episodes at other times where he looks at things and feels they are not there, as if "no fine tuning" in his brain, "not quite with it"; with a buzzing in the ears and a sensation as if not being in the world (2).

Inability to concentrate (2), especially in a conversation.

Had used a little marijuana in the past.

A weak feeling.

Mild headaches.

Gets episodes where the above symptoms are more severe, with a swelling of the lymphatic glands.

Sleeps 12 to 14 hours per day (2).

Feels depressed, a despair about his fatigue. Some days he feels good; some days bad.

Is anxious (2) about whether he's going to get better.

He is an English teacher, but now teaches only nine hours per week.

Naps in the middle of the day; worse before 3 p.m.(2); better after 5 p.m.

Has allergies (2); hay fever, ragweed; mucus, mainly postnasal drip.

(He is intellectual, and it is hard to get symptoms or modalities.)

Has been training since age 12. Was always very healthy, "Joe athlete."

He is single, but usually has long-term relationships; has been with current partner for two years but doesn't want to get married.

No stress now. Is a sessional lecturer at a university.

Craves dairy (2), cereals (2), fruit (2), and ice cream (2). Eats little meat or salt. Used to love eggs; stopped eating them 1 1/2 years ago. Feels better with light salads.

Thirst is low; mainly for orange juice.

Sleeps well. Has to have eight hours of sleep; wakes unrefreshed (2).

A high sex desire.

(Somewhat confused about symptoms and jumps back to other symptoms.)

He was hit by a car seven years ago. Also fell down a cliff five years ago; suffered a broken ankle and compression fracture in the lower back.

Is sensitive to cold (3). Aggravated by cold air (3).

Character:
- "Easy to get along with."
- Disciplined. Once he decides to do something, he does it.
- Since Epstein-Barr, his self-confidence is down (2).
- Withdrawing; too tired to deal with people; feels as if he's acting with people.
- Running was a bolster to his self-confidence, and now he can't do it.

In the past, he would sometimes take antibiotics for colds; would always take them when he had a sore throat. Has had most vaccines without noticeable side effects. Lately, no colds.

Timid.

Family History:
- Mother: allergies; serious immune system problems; now on steroids.
- Father: healthy.
- Other family history unknown.

(We had a long discussion about homeopathy. He's very skeptical.)

Analysis of Case Number 2

The symptoms in this case were even less clear than those in the first case. In totality, the symptoms give us hints of a number of polycrests, but none very clearly. I decided to choose one from this hazy list: Silicea (one 200c dose).

The major reasons for this choice were as follows:

- Easy-going nature.
- Sensitivity to cold.
- Fatigue, easy exhaustion.
- Symptoms resulting from exposure to cold after sweating.

Plan: Silicea 200c.

Follow-Up on Case Number 2

First Follow-up: Six Weeks After the Initial Visit

He doesn't feel much better.

His energy level is a little better; able to do more physical activity.

Feels less fatigue (2).

Can do more physically.

Dizziness (1) is better.

The inability to concentrate is slowly improving.

Today, he has a cold; caught it after windsurfing in the cold.

Needs less sleep.

Food cravings are the same.

Sensitivity to cold is the same. Aggravation from the cold is the same.

(He is very skeptical. Even after relating the improved symptoms, he doesn't feel he's better and requires a very long discussion and explanation of homeopathy.)

No aggravation.

No new symptoms.

Has buzzing in his ears and floaters across his eyes (1).

Assessment: His energy level is better (fatigue improved), his concentration is better, and other chief symptoms are improved. So, waiting is in order, despite his reluctance to say he feels better.

Plan: Wait

(I am including further follow-ups in this case because they represent a common dilemma: The patient says he is no better, but the symptoms reveal a different story. We must exercise caution and allow time to pass before pronouncing this a cure.)

Phone Call: One Day Following the First Follow-Up

His cold is worse; started antibiotics today, with Contact C. Has green mucus and congestion. The mucus discharge is thick; previously, it was profuse and ran like a tap.

Thirstless; feverish.

Assessment: I decided to give Pulsatilla 30c because of its complementary nature to Silicea, which seemed to have helped him.

Plan: 1. Take Pulsatilla 30c as needed.
2. Go back to Silicea after cold resolves.
3. Stop all allopathic medications.

Warren Metzler: I do not understand why you would even consider prescribing anything other than a higher dose of the same remedy. What is the basis for the assumption that an acute illness appearing under constitutional treatment could ever require anything other than a higher dose of the same remedy?

Klein: Yes, there is a school of thought that says that in an acute situation one should stick with the same remedy. There is also a school of thought that says one should give a complementary acute remedy. And, in my experience, there is no one right way. Each office visit is unique. There is no one rule that covers every possible situation. Flexibility is my byword.

Second Follow-Up: Two Months After the First Follow-Up

He is about the same; up and down.

Still feels he has a "virus."

Feels fatigue (2), which is worse at the end of the day (2), around 3 p.m., and in the morning after rising (1).

Dizziness (2), with buzzing in the ears; is worse when walking fast (2).

Inability to concentrate.

He went hiking for five to six days.

Has recovered from his cold but is not dramatically better after the remedy.

Feels unwell. He doesn't have his normal edge; is bothered by the buzzing in his ears (2) and the floaters in his eyes.

This is his first day back to teaching.

His problems are "cyclical"; he feels he demands a lot of himself.

If he does a normal amount of exercise, he gets very tired.

At first, he felt "Why me?" Still feels this way.

Craves ice cream (2) and dairy (2).

Was trying an allergy/elimination diet.

Sleep is good.

Assessment: I note that he waited a long time before returning to the office or contacting me. This tells me he is still skeptical and that perhaps the remedies have not touched him very deeply.

Silicea helped him previously, but its action was probably disrupted by the acute episode (cold). So, I decided to give it another chance before changing remedies.

Plan: Silicea 200c.

Phone Call: One Month After the Second Dose of Silicea

No change at all. His fatigue and all other symptoms are the same. He wants to give up homeopathic treatment.

Assessment: At this point I decided to change remedies, something that perhaps is controversial for some of you. Why did I change? I did it because the patient was decidedly unimproved after a repeat of the remedy and because, if this were truly a Silicea patient, he would not have displayed so much health anxiety, aggressiveness, and skepticism. I find that Silicea patients can get anxious but usually only in a very acute situation such as asthma. Usually, their anxiety has to be drawn out of them through questioning because they are so yielding.

After some thought, I decided to review the case and give the back-up remedy I had chosen, Scutellaria lateriflora 200c. The patient refused to return to the office because he was so skeptical. So, I had one more try, over the phone.

Plan: Scutellaria lateriflora 200c.

Third Follow-Up: Two Months After the Scutellaria

"Doing very well, definitely 95 percent better." Feels "reborn."

He is doing things he could not do before. Right after the remedy, he noticed a definite improvement.

No aggravation.

General, as well as specific, improvement.

The dizziness, buzzing, and inability to concentrate are completely gone.

Has no fatigue; started exercising again.

Is sleeping eight hours per day.

No allergies.

Is still sensitive to cold (2); avoids cold.

Craves ice cream (3) and dairy (2).

The disorientation is gone.

Assessment: He is better and, despite a lack of aggravation, he has been remarkably better for two months. Note that he decided to return again to the office for the follow-up.

It is hard to say that this is coincidence or that Silicea finally "clicked in," because he noticed this change right after the Scutellaria was administered. From experience, I believe that, if I had given Scutellaria as the first prescription, it would have worked well. Scutellaria was the correct first prescription. The Silicea was close enough to affect the vital force, to give a "glancing effect," but it did not last and was not really that exact simillimum we are looking for. Look carefully at the Silicea follow-up, and you will see the dissatisfaction with the efficacy of the initial prescription, both in my mind and in the patient's mind. The Scutellaria, on the other hand, brought about a profound change.

This case, unfortunately, brings up a point that I have found problematic. When I hear a new prescriber who has practiced for one or two years say, "I am getting 95 percent results with my cases," I wonder if he or she is getting the kind of results that Silicea produced in this case.

A related problem is when other practitioners state that they are using a kind of "zig-zag" approach to prescribing, whereby they give one remedy that has a slight effect, quickly switch to another one, and so on, and then say they all worked. I did not switch from Silicea lightly; it required a lot of thought. When I did switch, I waited to make sure that the Scutellaria would work in a deep way.

This is not to say that certain cases are not one-sided, as Hahnemann stated. On the other hand, we have to be clear and honest about what is working and what is not working in order to advance our prescribing skills.

Plan: Wait.

Long-Term Follow-Up

It has been three years, and this patient has been well without another remedy.

A Discussion of Scutellaria Lateriflora

Scutellaria lateriflora, common name skullcap, is an increasingly important remedy for use by modern homeopaths. Unfortunately, information in materia medicas and repertories is scanty. It is in only 18 rubrics in Kent's repertory, as plain-type references. Eleven of these symptoms refer to head pains. The provings have been done with the tincture, so they offer little of a refined or subtle nature with peculiar modalities. Probably the most useful information I have found is in Boericke's materia medica, from which I quoted in the first case.

In developing the beginnings of a "picture" of this remedy, I have worked backwards from cured clinical cases (some cases are not included here). Also, much of the proving, repertory, and materia medica information has helped me to form an initial understanding of the essential nature of a Scutellaria set of symptoms. This remedy picture suggests the remedy's particular usefulness in post-influenzal-type syndromes.

The provings discuss an "inability to study, stupor, confusion on studying," with an accompanying dull headache. In my experience, Scutellaria patients will say that they feel a sense of confusion and will describe it variously as being "off-balance," "off-center," or "dizzy." When you attempt to confirm whether it is a true vertigo, you find out that it isn't. It is not a profound vertigo, but rather a sensation that the world is not experienced clearly. They may describe this as "not being in the world" or "as if reality is askew." It can also be accompanied by depth perception problems. This state follows an acute influenza.

With this sensation and/or altered perception comes a ringing in the ears (without ear pathology), an inability to concentrate, and feelings of nausea, low vitality, and weakness. This sensation also leads to anxiety, an unexpressed resentment, and a feeling of injustice (although they are not bitter people).

The anxiety is low level and at times reaches a more profound intensity, a "nervous fear" as Boericke describes it. It is not expressed to others around them and they do not want others to see their condition. Rather, to others, they will simply say they are profoundly tired and need to sleep a lot. They become very sensitive to stimuli, such as noise or noisy places with lots of action, so they withdraw from their normal activities.

They then develop a more profound anxiety about accomplishing tasks and about the future. They feel that something terrible is going to happen. They worry about being able to function. Unlike Calcarea carbonica, this worry is associated with an underlying nervous, off-balance sensation, especially when in public or trying to concentrate. There is a quiet restlessness that accompanies the anxiety, but these people have little energy to expend the restlessness and tend to continue to keep to themselves. They become sleepless, restless and worried at night, and have night terrors, but definitely not as profound as in Stramonium.

The resentment I mentioned is a feeling of injustice about their state of health or how much work they have to do even though they feel ill. They often will talk of injustices, having sensitivities similar to Causticum, but are too weak to follow through and never develop the extreme revolutionary nature of Causticum.

The headaches, in my experience, are frontal, and the patient will refer to them as sinus headaches. Patients state that the headaches "weigh down the whole of the face" and are pressing in nature. Occasionally, these headaches extend back over the whole head. They complain about a headache after too much activity or excitement. Accompanying the headache is the sensorial confusion, as above, an inability to concentrate, and sleepiness during the day.

Scutellaria patients experience a frustration about their health, but when they express their symptoms during the interview, they ramble and the words to describe their condition don't come to mind. They can easily carry on other conversations that are not about their health. They express their symptoms in a confused way, moving back to symptoms previously expressed and trying unsuccessfully to explain them clearly. While you are taking the case, it is very hard to confirm their symptoms or get a clear idea of what they are trying to express.

They will also question your ability to help them. They will not question your personal abilities. Rather, they are questioning homeopathy itself. You will get an impression of sweetness and friendliness from them, rather than a feeling of intensity. Although, if you don't help them, they get more aggressive and skeptical of homeopathy. They also do not give much out in an emotional sense. You do not get the impression that they are sympathetic, rather that they are self-focused.

Other important components of Scutellaria are as follows:

- Chilly, or sensitive to heat, or sensitive to heat and cold; get chilled easily and have complaints from being chilled.

- Nausea, gas, and distention without modalities.

- To be thought of in post-influenzal cases, where there are few symptoms and modalities except mild anxiety. These are cases where it is hard to feel very confident about other remedies or even the Scutellaria prescription.

- Their complaints are continuous, but can get worse, and then they intermittently describe it as having the flu.

As you can see from my description of Scutellaria, many different remedies come to mind, especially with regard to certain symptoms or sets of symptoms. The difference is that, with a polycrest or a remedy used more frequently, we see more general confirmatory symptoms or stronger "essence" information than with a Scutellaria case.

In general, when there is a paucity of symptoms, we think either of a miasmatic remedy or of a minor remedy that is more specific to the situation. Scutellaria is the remedy to think of and use where there has been a history of recurrent flus and sinus infections with antibiotics frequently prescribed.

Scutellaria compares with other "post-influenzal" remedies, such as:

- Influenzinum (post-influenzal, paucity of symptoms)
- Gelsemium (anxiety, post-influenzal, frontal headache)
- Silicea (as in the second case)
- Bryonia
- Natrum salicylicum (post-influenzal prostration, tinnitus, Meniere's disease)
- Sulphur
- Natrum muriaticum
- Medorrhinum
- Cypripedium pubescens
- Causticum
- Baptisia

Obviously, this list is not complete. There is not time in this presentation to compare each of the above remedies with Scutellaria. It would be a good idea, though, to review the main points of Scutellaria and compare them with the main points of each of these and other such remedies in their post-influenzal phase. (The symptoms in parentheses do not represent these main points; they are just a few very brief notes.)

[The speaker asked the prescribers in the audience for their experiences with remedies useful for post-influenzal fatigue syndromes. Suggestions included Ferrum metallicum, Carbo vegetabilis, Carbo animalis, and Phosphorus. Other suggestions are as follows.]

Jeff Baker: I have two cured cases of long-standing chronic fatigue syndrome in which Eupatorium perfoliatum was the remedy. In both cases there was marked leukopenia, and both patients responded very well.

Klein: What were the guiding symptoms of those cases? Do you remember?

Jeff Baker: There were chronic remittent episodes of the flu-like symptoms — high fever, vomiting, and other symptoms. But it was the characteristic aching in the bones, as if they would break, that led me to prescribe Eupatorium perfoliatum. Both patients recovered completely.

Klein: Very interesting cases.

Audience: I work with a very skilled homeopath. He says that Scutellaria and Kali phosphoricum are the two main remedies for post-influenzal problems.

Klein: Yes, Kali phosphoricum is very similar to Silicea. Kali phosphoricum patients have a very low self-confidence because they make a lot of mistakes. They have trouble concentrating. You think of it where someone has been doing a lot of mental work and becomes very depleted, and then gets the flu and becomes even more depleted.

Scutellaria may also be compared generally to other polycrests and smaller remedies, such as:

- Calcarea carbonica (anxiety, anxiety about the future)
- Calcarea sulphurica (weakness, post infections)

- Psorinum (weakness, despair, anxiety)
- Alumina (confusion)
- Alumina silicata (very profound confusion and weakness)
- Lycopodium clavatum (anxiety, anxiety in regard to work)
- Argentum nitricum (anxiety, anxiety with vertigo-like perceptions)
- Arsenicum album (chilly, weakness, anxiety)
- Thuja (confusion in relating the case, paucity of symptoms, skepticism)
- Silicea (weakness, timidity)
- Mercurius (weakness, anxiety, salivation, sensitivity to heat and cold)
- Cannabis indica (sensorial affections)

I want to make a few additional comments about Argentum nitricum in this context. You may have noticed that there were some elements of Argentum nitricum in Case Number 1. I have noted that many Argentum nitricum individuals come in for treatment after the flu, which in itself is interesting.

You will see a continuum of Argentum nitricum symptoms. They needed Argentum nitricum before the flu, and they still need it afterwards. These people, as you know, are normally very warm-blooded. But after the flu, they will become quite chilly and actually have chills. Yet their post-influenzal symptoms will still indicate the need for Argentum nitricum.

It is important to understand as thoroughly as possible the patient's state of health before the flu in order to understand the ongoing stresses and the patient's response to these stresses.

Again, with the major (polycrest) remedies, you are going to be able to perceive and get many more confirmatory symptoms, a more extensive and stronger history, than you will with Scutellaria. The symptoms, then, will justify prescribing a polycrest remedy that runs through both the current post-influenzal condition and the pre-existing condition. The confirmatory symptoms or essence of the case will be strong.

With a Scutellaria case, the pre-existing symptoms are not strong or compelling for prescribing purposes. The strong points, in terms of what you can base your prescription on, are in the post-influenzal syndrome, off-center vertigo sensation, anxieties, nausea, weakness, dull frontal headache as if weighing down the face, and sleeplessness with fear — all of which will take you to Scutellaria.

This information on Scutellaria is incomplete, as is true with all of our remedies, especially the minor ones. It's waiting for your experience. I hope you will share with me any of your Scutellaria cases. That way, we can continue to expand our knowledge together.

Case Number 3

Let's look at another post-influenzal case. I am including this case in my presentation for comparison and interest. It is my earnest hope that it will help you develop an important attribute as a classical prescriber: flexibility. Specifically, it is important to develop the flexibility to understand the fluid nature of a remedy's essential features or essence so that you can prescribe it in many different situations that call for it. With this understanding you must remember that, for purposes of analysis, the picture of the whole person takes precedence over the particular symptoms and specific disease conditions.

I would also add that, although we use much of the general emotional information from the patient for evaluation purposes, we want to see some real and profound shifts in the patient's chief complaint or specific condition at the follow-up, and not just "psychological adjustments!" This rigorous approach, and the resultant curative results, will promote homeopathy to the forefront of medicine.

The case is a long and interesting one.

Female
Age 45
Bus Driver and Writer

Initial Visit

She has suffered from canker sores in her mouth (2) for the past 25 years; anywhere in the mouth, even in the throat. They are painful and annoying. Diagnosed (by naturopaths) as an allergy to mercury in fillings and high acidity. Worse after getting fillings; metallic taste (2) with the sores.

Her stomach is acidic (2); worse after eating tomatoes.

Constipation (2); anal fissures (2).

Has all of her father's problems.

Tired (3); no energy two to three hours after rising; worse at 12 noon (2); lifts weights and swims every day, but then tired.

Has been off work for two months. Had the flu, then a middle ear imbalance (now better); chronic fatigue; EEG was done.

She contracted the flu three months ago. Felt "really beat"; sweating, cold, and very irritable; averse to anything touching her.

Is asleep by 10:30 to 11 p.m.; sleeps through the night.

Was on an allergy diet for 20 days; the diet has been erratic since allergy testing; uses protein, a fiber supplement, and Herbatox.

Drives a bus:
- Works three-month shifts.
- Drives from Vancouver to Ladner, six times per day.
- Fears the tunnel (2); buses are too wide; no room in the tunnel to play.
- Too many variables; becomes tense (2).
- Unrealistic schedule; always running late, then getting angry (2).
- Frustrated (2).
- No recourse.
- An exercise in frustration; left with the feeling that you are a number in the system.
- Strives to get passengers to their destinations on time.
- No one in the system cares.
- Received 15 commendations in a year; company has to send letter, but they really don't care.
- Has worked there for two years.
- Impersonal nature of the work; likes the work but not the system.

She is a writer. She took the bus driving job to allow time to write; actually, puts in a 12-hour day. Wants to be at work; likes work; enjoys work. Work consumes too much energy. Writing a book and not enough time for it.

She has two children, 18 and 20 years old. Her 18-year-old daughter lives by herself; is a "hippie"; doing grade 12. Her 20-year-old son is a "yuppie"; he's living with the patient.

She has been in a relationship with a man for the past 1 1/2 years, which is a source of frustration, disappointment, anger, and hurt:
- Won't see him for months at a time.
- A struggle that he is the way he is.
- Is angry at herself (3) when she isn't recognized.
- Feels angry resignation; doesn't strive for anything.
- He's married; "He's not who I want him to be."
- Is upset when he doesn't call.
- They separate after an argument.

(getting excited)

Gets angry easily (2). "I'm a powerful person; I kill people verbally, so people don't screw around with me. If you cross this barrier, then you die."

"I haven't met anyone who is as aware as I am. People are in a stupor."

Has an adversarial side (2); others are going to lose.

She and her husband were together for 16 years. She decided to leave. She was Catholic, and it was hard to leave. She felt duty-bound. It took her four years to get out. Her ex-husband remarried; the children stayed with her.

She won't bother to get married; likes time alone (3).

Her sex desire is okay; sex doesn't drive her.

She always pushes through what she's afraid of. Is terrified on boats, but pushes through to gain respect for herself.

Is into personal growth seminars; many "profound changes" after one such seminar.

Character:
- People person; takes care of people.
- Dark side (1).
- "Superior" attitude (3), but not in the bus. This attitude comes out when she feels threatened.
- If others try to get the better of her, "You don't pull that on me."
- Friends know she's straight, but never cruel with people.
- Avoids hurting others' feelings (2); sulks if her feelings are hurt (2).

- Impression is that she's "alive."
- Loves everything when things are working right (2); then, "I'm the greatest person to be with."
- Does not want support (2); withdraws (2) when hurt.
- Averse to consolation (3); "It's a waste of time, not useful."

Family History:
- Father: died in 1982 at age 67, of a heart attack; the patient grieved (almost weeping).
- Mother: died at age 54 of cancer of the uterus.

When she can't achieve, she doesn't feel good. "I can master anything." Expects a lot from herself and others (3). Gets disappointed.

(sighs)

Her best friend died of an aneurysm when the patient was 16; this put the patient face to face with mortality. She felt abandoned by her friend; she is still angry and cries thinking about her. After the death, the patient was very upset; she wouldn't go to the same school, and was sent to a boarding school.

Felt grief when she couldn't stay married; made the decision and then fait accompli; all grief was over.

Fears that others will leave her.

Craves chocolate (3), milk, pasta (1), fish, and bananas (2).

Averse to spicy, meat, and acidic foods. Doesn't eat meat or chicken. Worse with spicy foods and tomatoes (2) (upsets stomach and causes heartburn).

Low thirst (2); forces herself to drink.

Is startled by loud noises.

Worries about brakes failing on a hill.

Is sensitive to cold (3) and irritable in heat (2); gets cold easily (2).

Has back pain (2); lower back and upper neck (1). Was in a motor vehicle accident in 1956; went through the windshield.

She's had three episodes of lesions on her cervix (2); the main symptom was very yellow urine, with a bitter smell (2).

Her menses are regular. Before menses, her sexual drive is higher (2), and her breasts are tender and sore (2).

She had blackouts eight times per day when she had the flu, but took no medications. The blackouts were sudden, lasted a short time (petit mal?), and affected her balance and short-term memory. They frightened her. She had thoughts of dying (2). "Maybe this is dying" (2).

As a child, she was exposed to fluorspar, lapis albus, and a radioactive water source. Her teeth are discolored, and she has a dry mouth.

She is sensitive to medications. Has a block about taking things; mistrusts medications.

Impression: As the interview progressed, she became more and more worked up and aggressive. At one point, she was very aggressive.

Analysis of Case Number 3

In this case, we see a post-influenzal complaint, but we have enough symptoms to prescribe a longer-term remedy on the basis of predisposing factors. If you take the emotional component of this case and attempt to analyze the information piece-meal, you may not see the forest for the trees. Based on small snippets of information, you may prescribe certain polycrests such as Natrum muriaticum, Ignatia, Sepia, and Sulphur.

However, it is important in this particular case to get an understanding of the whole case, including the way this woman related her symptoms and the "pace" of the case. Kent recommends that we get an understanding of the characteristics of each symptom by judging them in the context of the whole of the case. By "pace," I mean that she gets quite worked up as the case progresses. At certain points she gets very worked up, both in terms of her anger and in terms of describing herself. She says things like, "I'm the greatest to be with." Taken alone, we can interpret these statements as egotism, but in the context of the way she gets worked up, what would you say it is? It is exaltation. In the repertory under "exaltation," it says "see exhilaration." Stramonium is in this rubric.

We have other indications for Stramonium. We see that anger is an overriding force for her. This anger and her manner in general are strongly aggressive, and the pathology is really on the mental level. There is also a fear of tunnels and boats (water, small enclosed places).

We must not forget the fatigue, worse at noon. Stramonium is in this rubric. Even in the rubric "sighing," we find Stramonium. I have found that, because our society accepts very high levels of violence, I am frequently prescribing Stramonium for a variety of conditions, with profoundly curative results.

Plan: Stramonium 200c, one dose.

First Follow-Up After Stramonium

"I feel better."

She had one episode of canker sores (1) (better); the canker sores are trying to come "but not worth making them."

Her tiredness is better.

She has been working at night until 1:30 a.m.; now has the energy to do this.

The constipation (2) is the same. Her stools are hard and big (2) and painful. Has anal fissures. Occasionally uses a suppository.

Is doing a lot of writing; is tapping into her creative energy; it is flowing more freely.

Still has back pain (1).

Has had tender, sore breasts before menses, but no symptoms before her last menses.

Her nails are growing.

Plan: Wait. No remedy.

I included this follow-up to demonstrate that, even though a large part of the analysis was based on emotional, "character-type" symptoms and symptoms from the past, the particular and general symptoms comprising her chief complaints also improved. The patient has continued to do very well.

In order for homeopathy to be truly effective, we must see it as a therapy encompassing all aspects of suffering, to be applied with great flexibility in each individual case.

David Taylor Reilly, MD

A CASE OF INTRACTABLE CLUSTER HEADACHES

David Taylor Reilly, MD, holds the Research Chair at the University Department of Medicine, Glasgow, Scotland, jointly sponsored by the British Government and the Research Council on Complementary Medicine. He is perhaps best known for his research in the treatment of hay fever and asthma with homeopathic medicine. His hay fever study appeared in the October 1986 issue of The Lancet.

Introduction

It is appropriate that this is a case conference. The treatment of individuals is the foundation of medicine. In a way, every consultation is a clinical trial that provides the raw material to drive all medicine forward.

Although we have made great strides as a community, statistics suggest that 97 percent of the people in the United Kingdom still do not have easy access to a specialist trained in homeopathic medicine. We have about 1,000 homeopaths for a population of 55 million in the United Kingdom. I feel this is still a dismally small number of homeopaths. My principal goal is to alter this situation in a positive way.

In trying to alter this situation, I am constantly conscious of the importance of language and of the necessity to use the correct terms in order to communicate effectively. In communications between traditional or complementary forms of medical practice and the dominant modern medical practice, the point of contact is the patient. The patient is the one element that we all have in common.

Therefore, I believe that the clinical setting can be the most powerful source of positive development. To confirm this belief, I asked over 200 general practitioners in Great Britain what sort of evidence they wanted before they would sanction the use of homeopathy or a complementary medicine on their patients. Was it laboratory evidence? Was it basic science? Was it clinical trials? The surprising information that emerged was that they placed a high priority on positive clinical results and on positive patient experiences. Of course, general practitioners really know in their hearts that it is clinical experience and responsive patients that ultimately determine where and how a treatment will be used. They also know that medicine is not a science. It is a myth that medicine is a science.

So, for all our divisions, the medical community is united by a desire to help our patients. For the last three years I have been working in the University Department of Medicine in Glasgow, exploring the boundaries between orthodox and alternative or complementary medicine. I have found that a thoughtful video case presentation is a powerful way to bridge the orthodox-heterodox gap. I have successfully used a seven-minute video of an interview with the patient in this case during 30-minute introductory presentations of homeopathy to orthodox medical audiences. I would like to present this case, not so much in the hope of teaching you homeopathy (I would not be so presumptuous), but rather to discuss the contact and the views such a bridge can make possible.

For 50 percent of my week I am a specialist in internal medicine, completely orthodox medicine. I do emergency receiving of patients in diabetic ketoacidosis, heart attacks, and other conditions, and I provide conventional outpatient care. For the other half of the week I conduct my complementary medical work. When my turn came to make a case presentation to my orthodox colleagues, I presented a homeopathic case. You could have cut the air with a knife [laughter]. I had 30 minutes in which to explain homeopathy, the case in question, and its response to homeopathic treatment. I realized as I did this that, in a way, it was a climax of a five-year apprenticeship in trying to communicate with such audiences.

The result of this case presentation was a three-month silence [laughter]. But after three months I was sent a case referral from another internal medical specialist who requested that a patient be treated with complementary medicine. This patient also had chronic headaches that did not respond to conventional treatments. I treated him with auricular acupuncture, and the pain has never returned.

This success prompted an increasing trickle of referrals. It has now reached the point that two complementary medicine clinics are run each week in the orthodox medicine department. One of them is with the anesthetists working in the pain clinic, and one is a general medical clinic. These clinics treat people who otherwise would not have had any exposure to complementary medicine.

The trust that this developed with my colleagues supported the development of research and educational programs. The postgraduate homeopathic course, for example, has grown to be the most vigorous postgraduate medical course in Scotland, attracting about 90 to 100 new doctors each academic year. It is now part of the official educational structure within the country.

I do believe in the value of talking to people. If we are outside the system (as we are), we can get angry, arrogant, and depressed. But what does that accomplish? The fact is, we have to knock on the door. It is not going to come to us.

The features of this case that I think are helpful to a questioning but skeptical audience include the following: a clear organic disease of general medical interest that has been investigated and diagnosed by experts; failure of comprehensive orthodox treatment to cure the disease; failure of acupuncture, which was given in the same therapeutic setting as the later homeopathy; no response to a single-blind prescription of a homeopathic placebo; and, finally, a clear and sustained response to homeopathic treatment.

Indeed, the case meets many of the criteria of an n=1 trial (Ref. 1). Further, the syndrome is an elegant starting point for a discussion in a common language about the modalities of signs and symptoms in disease, the empiricism of much medical treatment, and the relationships among therapies, toxicity, and the pathophysiology of disease. The only drawback is that the video-taped interview with the patient is in "Glaswegian" [laughter]. I have therefore included a full text of the interview later in my case presentation notes.

Cluster Headaches

This patient suffered from cluster headaches. I think it will enhance the understanding of the case if I precede the case presentation with brief details about cluster headaches, taken mainly from the *Oxford Textbook of Medicine (Ref. 2)*.

Also called migrainous neuralgia, Harris's syndrome, or Horton's syndrome, this curious syndrome mainly affects males 20 to 50 years old. It presents in the following ways.

Principal Features

Pain in the orbit of the eye, extending to the forehead, temple, cheek, and jaw. The pain is unilateral, of great severity, and comes in daily bouts of 30 to 120 minutes.

Usually occur at night, one hour after falling asleep, with "alarm-clock" regularity.

Occur in "clusters," lasting from 4 to 16 weeks, then remit completely until the next relapse. Occasionally (as in this case), the attacks continue for one year or more: "chronic migrainous neuralgia."

Associated Features

Eye: red, bloodshot, with profuse watering.

Nostril: blocked or running.

Horner's syndrome: one in four cases, occasionally persists.

Restlessness: "betrays the frightening severity"; pacing and night walks.

Precipitation: usually unknown; occasionally by alcohol and vasodilators. Precipitation by GTN (nitrates) can be diagnostic.

Remissions: complete between attacks.

Etiology

The etiology is unknown. There is a rise in histamine during attacks, but its significance is unknown. There is an autonomic involvement as shown by the occurrence of the Horner's syndrome. Carotid syphon edema has been noted. It is very rare to have migraines also; the syndrome is associated with peptic ulceration.

Diagnostic Investigations

Investigations are not necessary because the presentation is so classical. Trigeminal neuralgia, migraines, and other cephalalgias may need to be considered as differential diagnoses, but the quality, timing, duration, and distribution of cluster headache symptoms are very characteristic.

Conventional Treatments

A number of powerful agents are used. Historically, some were employed empirically. From a homeopathic perspective, it is interesting that the two main treatments can also cause severe headaches.

Ergotamine: taken one hour in anticipation of an attack and before bed, as suppositories, inhaler, or subcutaneous; use six days and test on seventh day. Maximum dosage is 12 mg per week; otherwise, there is a risk of ergotism. Withdrawal from Ergotamine may cause rebound headaches.

Methysergide: an antiserotonin drug. Dosage of 1 to 2 mg, three per day, for a maximum of six months, watching for side effects of fibrosis, arterial spasm, and edema. Methysergide must be stopped gradually to avoid rebound headaches.

Pizotifen: "anti-biogenic amines," less effective.

Lithium: "mechanism unknown," for use in chronic cases if other therapies fail. Side effects include nephrogenic diabetes insipidus, central nervous system problems, and thyroid dysfunction.

Other Treatments: In intractable cases, there may be recourse to steroids, oxygen, and stellate ganglion blocks.

Case History

This case history is taken from the presentation in August 1986, when the patient was referred by his general practitioner to the acupuncture clinic of the Glasgow Homoeopathic Hospital.

Because this case has been used to introduce homeopathy to orthodox academic audiences, I have left the information in the form used on these occasions. It is followed by the full text of an interview, which allows the patient to speak for himself.

Mr. R. McK.
Born: March 10, 1951

Social History

The patient is a plumber by trade. He is married; his wife has a son by a previous marriage. He is sterile, and AIDS is being considered. He smokes 20 cigarettes per day; has not had alcohol since a minor hematemesis. He breeds budgies and has not worked since 1984 because of illness. In 1986, his wife gave up her job and applied for an attendance allowance to look after him.

Medical History

- 1976: Abdominal testicle removed. (Precipitated the clusters?)
- 1979: Bone graft in right wrist.

- 1984: Bornholm's disease.
- A number of traumatic fractures.

Presenting Problem: The Main Symptoms

- "Intractable" chronic migrainous neuralgia: cluster headaches.
- Started in 1976; classical features, except that the headaches are not remitting.
- Three 90-minute attacks per day.
- Right-sided, extremely severe facial pain.
- Associated with swelling of the palate and face on the affected side.
- Red eye; discharge from right eye and nostril.
- Went blind on three occasions.
- Nosebleeds occasionally precede the attacks.
- Vomiting.

Diagnostic Investigations

- Routine ++++
- VDRL/TPHA
- RF/ANF: negative
- X-ray of sinuses and chest
- Dental x-rays
- Angiogram
- Two CT Scans

Treatment Summary

Pizotifen (Sanomigran)	1983
Methysergide (Deseril)	1984
Prednisolone	1984
Nefedipine (Adalat)	1984
Ergotamine (Medihaler)	1984
Prochlorperazine (Stemetil)	1984
Dihydrocodeine (DF118)	1984
Co-proxamol (Disalgesic); 20/day!	1984
Lithium carbonate	1985
Lithium and methysergide	1985
Carbemazepine (Tegretol)	1986
Buprenorphine (Temgesic)	1986
Cyproheptadine (Periactin)	1986

- Dental plates   1985
- Stellate ganglion block   1985
- Caffeine-free diet   1985

Progress

September 1983 — dental hospital:
- Received a prescription of Pizotifen, from a neurologist.

December 1983 — neurological institute:
- "Thirty-two-year-old; six years of intermittent right facial pain.
- Diagnosis: migrainous neuralgia."
- Prescription: Methysergide; initial response, but failed on second course.

By October 1984:
- Prescription: Prednisolone and emergency admissions; no response.
- Prescription: Nefedipine; no response.
- "Impressed with description of cluster headaches with lacrimation; palate and facial swelling."
- Prescription: Ergotamine and Dihydrocodeine (IM); short-lived response (two weeks).
- Prescription: Methysergide; no response.
- Rhinorrhea; pain for hours.
- Suicidal; eager to accept stellate ganglion block.

March 1985:
- Second CT scan.
- Stellate ganglion block for Horner's syndrome, but no relief.
- Prescriptions: Lithium carbonate and Methysergide; caused confusion, hallucinations, and ataxia at first. Settled, with some reduction in symptoms. Despite possible side effects (muscle and urinary pain), he is not willing to stop the prescription.

July 1985:
- Taken off of Methysergide; maintains reasonable control on Lithium and Dihydrocodeine.

November 1985:
- Still reasonable control; facial pain. Dentist's prescription seems to aggravate the problem.

May 1986:
- Continued chronic problem; deteriorating condition.
- Prescription: Carbemazepine, needing increasing Buprenorphine.

June 1986:
- Wife seeks attendance allowance; very poor pain control.
- Prescription: Cyroheptadine (Periactin).
- General practitioner: "Only morphine left." Sends patient to the homeopathic hospital for acupuncture.

Homeopathic Hospital

July 1986:
- Two months of acupuncture and counseling; little response.

August 1986:
- In-patient observation.
- Prescription: Single-blind placebo; no response.
- Prescription: Active homeopathic drug, 10M potency; instant positive response (within seconds), with one week of increased frequency of clusters, each responding to the drug, then complete remission.
- Stopped all other treatments.

November 1986:
- Mild recurrence (one day); responds to three doses of the same homeopathic drug.

June 1987:
- Single headache; responds to same homeopathic drug.

March 1988:
- Nineteen months of remission; no other prescription is required.
- "I'm frightened because I feel so well. I keep expecting a relapse."

Update

November 1989: 2 1/2 years of remission. Following a series of extremely stressful personal and family crises, he relapses with a dominant element of anxiety and depression. Restarts smoking; drinks 20 to 30 cups of tea per day. He responds to the homeopathic drug. The response is less dramatic than previous responses, however, and he requires counseling, practical advice, and a homeopathic prescription for his depression. His condition settles in four weeks.

Patient Interview

This interview was taped in November 1986, five months after treatment.

Doctor: Robert is a 36-year-old man whom we first saw about five months ago. You presented initially to the acupuncture clinic, where you had been referred to me by your general practitioner. The story was of right-sided cluster headaches of 11 years' duration.

I'll just summarize the treatment you had had up until then. You had seen a lot of doctors and you had been to a lot of departments, hadn't you? Among other things, you have had Adalat, Methysergide, Ergotamine, DF118, Temgesic, Parlodel, steroids, Tegretol, and then Lithium. Anything else that we have missed out?

Patient: Probably will be, but I can't remember them all.

Doctor: It is enough to get on with. You've also been to your dentist who tried to fit in a special plate. I then started to treat you with some acupuncture, and, curiously, the first thing we did was to swap the problem.

Patient: That's right. It shifted from one side to the other.

Doctor: From the right to the other side, and it felt more or less identical on the opposite side, and then it returned to the original side. We weren't getting anywhere with the acupuncture, and I admitted you to the hospital for homeopathy. That's the basic background, but would you like to describe it from your own point of view — how the trouble started and what the symptoms felt like?

Patient: It starts like toothache. To me, it is toothache actually. Gradually it works its way into my jawbone and it just explodes in my head. You feel as if your head is going to explode wide open with the pain. It's that bad.

Doctor: What happens then?

Patient: My eye runs, my right eye goes pinky color, my nose runs, sometimes it actually bleeds. If I can get something to take the pain away it all clears up.

Doctor: Any other feelings or symptoms that are occurring in yourself during that time, in your general feelings, or any other changes in yourself?

Patient: I feel right down (depressed) or low.

Doctor: What sort of things can bring the trouble on?

Patient: I have never been able to draw any specific thing that I'm eating to cause it. Never ever could. And the hospitals stopped me drinking tea and taking chips and different things but it never made any difference.

Doctor: I remember the first time I saw you. You were really different then. You were really down at that time. You said something about your concentration. Can you remember that?

Patient: It was hard to focus on things.

Doctor: Has that any bearing on the headaches or not?

Patient: I don't really think so.

Doctor: I think, at that time, when you mentally concentrated, your pain could get worse. Is that true?

Patient: Yes, that's still the same, I feel.

Doctor: Can you describe what you would do during one of these episodes? How would you try to help or relieve yourself? What would you look like during one?

Patient: Somebody that is crazy. I've got to walk about. I cannot sit down or go into a darkened room and lie down. I've got to be walking about all the time. I find in the house I've got a blue bathroom suite, and being in that toilet seems to help the pain. It doesn't take the pain away but it stops it being as severe. The walking is the main thing.

Doctor: Does anything locally help? Cold or heat or pressure?

Patient: Well, the toilet is cold, so I don't know if maybe it's the coldness or the blue suite. I definitely like it in the toilet.

Doctor: There was some relationship to sneezing, I think.

Patient: When I take a headache, I cannot sneeze. When I try to sneeze, the sneeze will not come. Previous to taking a headache I try and I cannot sneeze. When I get that feeling, I know that the headache is going to come on.

Doctor: Would it be at any particular time of day or night?

Patient: It just comes on when it wants to come on.

Doctor: From what you were describing, when they come, do they come suddenly, or is it a gradual onset?

Patient: No, you don't get any warning. It just hits you.

Doctor: Could that literally be over seconds?

Patient: Oh, yes. It's been described to me as a nerve strangling a blood vessel in the brain... and when I take the pain in my teeth, this is the nerve reacting, and when it hits my head, this is the blood getting released and rushing to the brain.

Doctor: What do you think of that explanation?

Patient: I don't know about medical; I just accept what they tell me.

Doctor: How would your wife or other people find you emotionally, or in terms of your behavior or mood during these episodes? How are you behaving in terms of other people?

Patient: Abrupt. My wife, she is trying to help me; she tells me to go into a dark room and to lie on the bed. I tell her these things don't work. I shout at her and all the rest of it. Many a time if I had the guts I would jump out of the window.

Doctor: Is your temper quite violent at that time?

Patient: Yes.

Doctor: Have you struck out, or...?

Patient: I have not actually hit anybody; I have punched the wall. I've hit my head against the wall; it has been that sore.

Doctor: It goes without saying, hearing you describe it. But when I first met you, you really were not coping. You were quite down.

Patient: Yes. It was getting the better of me.

Doctor: Can you recall a little bit, how you viewed things at that time?

Patient: I felt myself... that something in my head was going to burst wide open. That I did. Even yet, although the powders are helping me, when I had that wee spot of headaches again it felt that my head would burst right open.

Doctor: You had actually...considered hurting yourself?

Patient: I'm too much of a coward.

Doctor: In between the actual headaches, were you still a bit irritable and down? How were you in between?

Patient: Before I started to take these powders, I slept all the time and was very impatient. Driving the car, in front of traffic lights (it wasn't the traffic lights' fault), I could not just sit and wait till they turned to green and I could go. Sometimes I had to jump them and I could not sit there.

Doctor: In what other ways were you showing that you were not yourself?

Patient: I was picking on my boy. He likes to play his records up loud. I was going in and telling him to get them off. He wasn't having any pals in because of the noise. Any wee thing I'd pick up, like, if my wife hadn't washed a cup, I'd jump down her throat.

Doctor: Was this placing a real strain on the relationship at home?

Patient: Oh, yes, our sex life was nonexistent.

Doctor: Was that because there was a loss of interest or feeling?

Patient: A loss of interest on my part. My wife approached me. I don't know why, but it wasn't there.

Doctor: Even on your own? Were there any feelings at any time on your own?

Patient: No, it was a complete blank in my mind.

Doctor: As well as obviously this irritability that you are describing and the feeling of downness, did you have any actual fears? Can you recall? Any specific worries?

Patient: I've got worries. Since I had an operation in my stomach 11 years ago when a testicle was removed I've not been able to father a child. And that's always preyed on my mind. My wife did actually fall pregnant 10 years ago; she had a threatened miscarriage. The hospital said that it (the fetus) was four months, but the possibility of the baby surviving was 50-50. So they made me make that decision inside half-an-hour, and they advised me to get it taken away, which I agreed. And now it's always on my mind that if I hadn't let them take it away maybe the wean (baby) would have survived. I do feel guilty about that.

I have been accepted on this artificial insemination list, but that's been hit on the head with this AIDS scare. I'm not going ahead with this now. My wife is maybe over-desperate to have a child, and I know that gets to me and I'm always frightened that if I cannot give her a child maybe she'll go elsewhere.

Doctor: And was that feeling preying on your mind around the time when I met you, or is this more a background?

Patient: I suppose it's always really there.

Doctor: I see. Okay. So... I well recall when we brought you into the hospital how down you were and how distressed you were. Do you want to describe what happened to you after you received treatment?

Patient: I was a new man altogether, absolutely fantastic after I had the powders.

Doctor: I remember we started you on one sort of medicine (placebo) and then swapped to a different sort (active). I don't know if you now recall that — the difference between the first few powders you had which didn't seem to work too much and then we changed them to another medicine and you were able to say right away.

Patient: Within seconds you could feel it working.

Doctor: What happened then with the first powder and then during the next few weeks?

Patient: The first powder (placebo) took about an hour or an hour and a half before it had an effect. It wasn't keeping the headaches away either.

Doctor: That was the very first medicine.

Patient: Yes.

Doctor: The second medicine.

Patient: You changed the powder. With the second medicine you could feel, within seconds of taking it, you could feel it working, taking the pain away from my teeth more or less instantly. But it took about a week before the headaches went away altogether.

Doctor: You were taking a powder with each headache at that time.

Patient: Yes.

Doctor: And then, after the first week, what happened in the weeks that followed?

Patient: It was fantastic. I felt like a new man. I hadn't felt as good since primary school. Fantastic.

Doctor: What sort of things did you notice were different about you as a person?

Patient: Well, it's difficult to explain. My wife is a person who likes to go out all the time. I just couldn't go out. I didn't have it in me to go out, but now I feel I want to go out and enjoy life. Before that, life just didn't exist.

Doctor: Until about two weeks ago, that's almost five months, I think I'm right in saying you were almost completely free of the headaches. Then, two weeks ago, you had a return of them. How did you handle things and what was it like?

Patient: They weren't as bad as they originally were. I believe that's because I took the powders right away.

Doctor: You went straight for them.

Patient: I was irritable again, irritable with my boy. I was getting on my wife's nerves. She even walked out on me one night. She came back right enough, but she just couldn't stand the way I was reacting.

Doctor: Was this shouting and...?

Patient: Yes. The least wee thing I was blowing up.

Doctor: And has that settled again?

Patient: Yes.

Doctor: How many powders did you have to use during the return of the symptoms?

Patient: Three powders.

Doctor: Was this by taking one dry and diluting the rest in water?

Patient: No, diluting them in water.

Doctor: Will you remind me why you decided to do it in that way. You noticed something yourself, didn't you?

Patient: I felt that when I was taking the powder dry on my tongue it wasn't doing anything. I tried it one night by taking it in water and I could feel it *reacting right away.*

Doctor: We advised you to take one dry, and then put the second one in water, and then to take a teaspoonful from the water.

Patient: Yes, that's right.

Doctor: Did you discover if it was the first dose in the water or did you need to repeat the medicine?

Patient: No, I've never had to repeat it.

Doctor: So, it's a single dose from the water and things start to settle?

Patient: Things go away after, at the most, five teaspoons from the water.

Doctor: Taking them how often?

Patient: Taking them every five minutes.

Doctor: Then, coming right up to date, the headaches have again disappeared. And how is your mood and your energy? Has it returned back to normal yet?

Patient: Everything's brighter.

Doctor: You told me before we started filming that you had a return of an older symptom.

Patient: Yes. Dizzy spells when I lie down and then get up. Everything is spinning. What's caused it I don't know. At the moment, I'm getting tablets from my doctor.

Doctor: Have you had this before in the past?

Patient: Years ago. My wife used to say it was because I was getting up too quick, and I always accepted that. I was getting up too quick. I know for a fact that this time it is nothing to do with getting up too quick. Even if I'm lying in bed and I shut my eyes, everything is spinning. So I can't blame it on getting up too quick this time.

Doctor: *How far do you have to go back before you can remember when it was last here?*

Patient: *It was a long time ago, before I got married actually, when I was about twenty.*

Doctor: *Okay. I think perhaps I don't need to prescribe for that, and I'll explain to you why in a moment. Thanks very much. Is there anything you want to add at the end, or have we covered things?*

Patient: *I feel that it's like a miracle what you've done for me.*

Case Analysis and Discussion

Reilly: *Would anyone like to suggest a prescription for this case?*

Audience: *Coffea cruda is a good possibility for pain in the teeth and for the symptom of having remorse.*

Reilly: *Right. Coffea is quite intolerant to pain.*

Audience: *Being simple-minded as I am, I would suggest Belladonna because of the right-sided headache and sudden onset.*

Reilly: *Right. It's a possibility. Anything else?*

Andrea Sullivan: *I would go along with Belladonna because it has a suicidal disposition, wanting to jump from a height. He talked about jumping out of the window from the pain. Also, he has rage and irritability with the headache. I also thought of Nux vomica, but I think I'd go with the Belladonna.*

Reilly: *Right. I was struggling at the time I saw this case between the idea of treating the patient and treating the disease. I sometimes therefore do a repertorization in two layers. We can look at the chronic (or intercurrent) condition between the headaches — the remorse, the suicidal disposition, the dwelling on past disagreeable events, and the withdrawal from company. I didn't point out earlier that he was completely impotent. A complete loss of any sexual desire was one of his symptoms. For the chronic state, I considered Natrum muriaticum. Then I decided to look at the local symptoms of the disease process. But now let me show you how I present this to an orthodox medical audience.*

Homeopathic Treatment

For those unfamiliar with this approach, I should explain that the object is to match the precise pattern of physiological disturbance in the patient to a homeopathic drug that will reproduce this problem in toxic doses. The homeopathic drug is then given in a subtoxic amount. This procedure is based on the empirical observation that actions at toxic and microdilutional levels are often opposite and antagonistic. Any further direct explanations are beyond the scope of this presentation, but you may wish to refer to an introductory article for further information (Ref. 3).

I approached the problem in two layers: the acute state and the intercurrent state. The two repertorizations included here (Kent's repertory on CARA, Version 4.6) give an idea of the homeopathic drugs I considered. You will note the highly individualized spectrum of symptoms and signs that homeopaths use.

Taking the repertorizations into account and bearing in mind that the condition has an autonomic element, I prescribed Belladonna 1M, wondering about Calcarea carbonica and Natrum muriaticum as second prescriptions. For over two years after Belladonna was given, no other remedy was needed. During the recent family crises/breakdown, Ignatia amara and Nux vomica were used without success. More Belladonna and emotional support ultimately proved successful.

The Materia Medica of Belladonna

Toxicology

In understanding why Belladonna was appropriate, it is interesting to begin by considering the conventional toxicology of this homeopathic drug, taken mainly from Martindale (Ref. 4). The principal side effects relate to the anticholinergic properties and are familiar to, and used by, those trained in homeopathy:

- Dry mouth, thirst, fewer secretions.
- Flushed face, erythematous rashes.
- Dilated pupils, photophobia, blurring, rise in intraocular pressure.
- Constipation, leading to ileus.

ACUTE PRESENTATION:

		Bell	Bry	Ars	Calc	Ign	Lach	Nux-vom	Con	Phos	Arg-n
PAIN-BURSTING	Head	***	***	*	***	*	***	—	***	***	*
PAIN-BURSTING,SO SEVERE UNBEARABLE	Head	—	—	*	***	—	—	—	—	—	—
PAIN-SUDDEN PAINS	Head	**	—	—	—	—	—	—	—	—	**
PAIN-SUDDEN,AND GO SUDDENLY	Head	**	—	—	—	**	—	—	—	—	—
PAIN-SIDE,RIGHT	Head	***	**	*	***	***	*	—	**	—	—
PAIN-EXTENDS TO HEAD	Teeth	—	**	*	*	—	—	*	—	*	—
PAIN-NEURALGIC	Teeth	***	—	—	—	—	—	—	—	—	—
PAIN-RIGHT	Teeth	***	**	—	**	—	*	**	—	*	—
LACHRYMATION-HEADACHE DURING	Eye	*	—	—	—	**	—	—	*	—	*
EPISTAXIS-HEADACHE,DURING	Nose	*	**	—	—	—	*	—	—	—	—
RESTLESSNESS-HEADACHE DURING	Mind	**	*	**	—	*	**	—	—	—	*
IRRITABILITY-HEADACHE,DURING	Mind	*	*	**	*	—	*	**	*	**	—
STRIKING-	Mind	***	—	—	—	**	—	**	—	*	—
STRIKING-HEAD AGAINST WALL	Mind	*	—	*	—	—	—	—	*	—	—
SUICIDAL-THROWING FROM HEIGHT	Mind	**	—	*	—	—	—	**	—	—	**

```
NUMBER OF RUBRICS MATCHED ->   13   7   7   6   6   6   5   5   5   5

TOTAL REMEDY SCORE ->          27  13   9  13  11   9   9   8   8   7
```

BACKGROUND STATE:

		Sulph	Hep	Nat-m	Lach	Plat	Bell	Carb-v	Nit-ac	Alum	Am-c
SADNESS-(Mental Depression)	Mind	***	**	***	***	***	**	**	***	**	**
SUICIDAL-(Disposition)	Mind	*	**	—	**	*	*	*	*	*	*
REMORSE	Mind	*	—	*	*	*	**	*	*	*	*
DWELLS-PAST DISAGREEABLE EVENTS	Mind	**	*	***	—	**	—	—	*	—	*
IRRITABILITY-TRIFLES	Mind	—	*	—	—	—	—	—	—	—	—
COMPANY-AVERSION	Mind	**	**	***	**	**	**	**	—	*	—
SEXUAL PASSION-WANTING	Male	**	*	**	*	—	*	**	**	*	*

```
NUMBER OF RUBRICS MATCHED ->    6   6   5   5   5   5   5   5   5   5

TOTAL REMEDY SCORE ->          11   9  12   9   9   8   8   8   6   6
```

- Urinary urgency, followed by retention.
- Hyperpyrexia, causing fatal heat stroke.
- Brady/tachycardia, arrhythmias.
- Excitation, leading to ataxia, delirium, and coma.

Homeopathic Trials (Provings)

Homeopathic human volunteer studies, using a range of concentrations, confirmed the above toxicology and expanded the prescribing data and precision by emphasizing functional disturbances occurring before gross toxicity.

The following notes, taken from standard homeopathic materia medicas (Ref. 5-7), give an idea of the homeopathic perception of Belladonna and show the striking correspondence between this patient's state and the Belladonna state.

In general, for SUDDEN ONSET - VIOLENT REACTIONS:

- Hyperaesthesia to touch, noise, and pain.
- Intense vascular congestion, especially of the head.
- Severe neuralgic pain coming and going suddenly in repeated attacks.
- Restlessness, excitation.

BELLADONNA HEADACHES are characterized by:

- Sudden onset, very intense.
- Vascular or neuralgic pains.
- Mainly right-sided.
- Throbbing in the head or teeth; "sensation as if the cranium would burst."
- Great restlessness; worse when lying down and from noise.
- Associated nasal congestion, nasal bleeding, and conjunctival congestion.

Clinical Use

Combining the homeopathic and toxicological data has led to the use of Belladonna in homeopathic dosage in a number of conditions, such as:

- Early infections/inflammations with suddenness, redness, and burning heat (such as boils, otitis media, and scarlet fever).
- Febrile convulsions and heat stroke.
- Intense colic.

- Acute headaches.
- Acute manias with visual hallucinations.

Closing Comments

In this particular case, the internally consistent correspondence between the clinical picture, the drug toxicology, and the response to treatment points to an underlying physiological correspondence. Conventional understanding of this disease suggests that there is an autonomic involvement. This understanding is reinforced by the response to Belladonna, which further suggests that the principal problem may be cholinergic regulation. I suspect that the homeopathic drug may be offering a signal for resetting system/receptor sensitivities, which it would have deranged at higher doses.

In any case, the divorce between homeopathic and orthodox wisdom helps no one, and a trial reconciliation seems in order. The contacts fostered by this and other individual cases have helped in establishing the current historic developments in complementary medicine in Glasgow University, including discussion seminars as a part of the undergraduate curriculum. I would like to record my gratitude to my patient and my respect for the importance of empirical clinical experience: the single case.

References

1. Guyatt G. et al. Determining optimal therapy — randomised trials in individual patients. *N Engl J Med*. 314 (1986): 889-892.

2. Weatherall D.J., J.G.G. Ledingham, D.A. Warrell (editors). *Oxford Textbook of Medicine*. 2nd Edition. Volume 2; Section 21.30. Oxford: Oxford University Press. 1987.

3. Reilly, D.T., and M.A. Taylor. The difficulty with homeopathy. *Complementary Medical Research* 3 (1988): 70-78.

4. Martindale. *The Extra Pharmacopoeia*. 28th edition. J.E.F. Reynolds (editor). London: The Pharmaceutical Press. 1982. Pp. 293-294.

5. Boericke, W. *Homoeopathic Materia Medica*. 9th Edition. London: Homoeopathic Book Services. Reprinted 1987. Pp. 110-115.

6. Phatak, S.R. *Materia Medica of Homoeopathic Medicines*. London: Foxlee-Vaughan Publishers. Reprinted 1988. Pp. 84-88.

7. Clarke, J.H. *A Dictionary of Practical Materia Medica*. London: The Homoeopathic Publishing Company. 1947. Pg. 260.

Notes on the Placebo Response

[Editors' Note: Dr. Reilly presented material from his clinical research on homeopathy and the placebo response. Because this material is not yet published, we have agreed to print only an abstract of the general points of this discussion.]

Doctors prescribe. Nature heals or kills. The placebo response would be better renamed a self-healing response; the nocebo response (negative action from placebos) would be better renamed a self-destructive response.

These responses are powerful. Intravenous saline injections can be as strong as morphine, and placebo cytotoxics have induced alopecia. Homeopathic practice is at least as capable of influencing this potential as any other form of medical intervention. How can we judge our treatment or add to our literature without a study of this area?

Much valuable work has already been done to identify some of the modifiers of these innate responses. These include the Interactive Triad:

- The patient's expectation of outcome.
- The clinician's expectation of outcome.
- The treatment effect.

Modified further by:

- The disease process.
- The treatment's form, route of administration, even color.
- The clinical setting.
- The cultural setting.

Homeopathy may act synergistically with self-healing responses and may therefore be modified by the factors known to affect the placebo response. The whole-system view of homeopathy preceded and still challenges recent developments in psychoneuroimmunology and the emerging mechanisms of mind-body interaction. Homeopathy has much to teach and to learn about this subject.

Reference:
Reilly, D.T. Homeopathy and Placebo — A Redundant Hypothesis?
Communications Br Hom Res Group. 1989. Pp. 121-131.

Peggy Chipkin, BS, RN, FNP

A CASE OF LEARNING DISABILITY IN AN ADOLESCENT BOY

Peggy Chipkin, BS, RN, FNP, graduated with a BS in Nursing from Cornell University and received her Family Nurse Practitioner training at the University of California at Davis. She has studied homeopathy since 1976, primarily with George Vithoulkas, Bill Gray, and Roger Morrison. Peggy is a founding member of the Hahnemann Medical Clinic, where she has practiced since 1985, and is an instructor in the Hahnemann College of Homeopathy, both in Berkeley, California.

A High IQ with Learning Disabilities

Initial Visit: October 7, 1989

The patient was a 15-year-old male. He had a normal build and was five feet, six inches tall.

The case was given by his mother:

Cannot learn (3); makes him feel worthless and depressed (2). Cannot comprehend the instructions; school has been like a torture all of his life.

Was considered "learning disabled" until a recent IQ test. IQ = 139.

Has been in some special education classes. Has problems with writing; composition, handwriting, and punctuation are all poor.

Sensitive (2). Teacher is very critical.

On a recent term paper assignment, every student except the patient followed the instructions accurately.

Is failing three courses this year.

Disorganized (2).

Absent-minded (2). Doesn't remember to take papers to school even when his mother puts them out and reminds him.

"Preoccupied" (2), as if he is far away; it is hard to have a conversation with him.

If under stress at school (i.e., doesn't know an answer) and his teacher pressures him, he says "I can't do it"(2) or rages (2). On a couple of occasions each school year, he would hold his head and run out of the room screaming. In grade school, he would lie on the floor holding his head, saying "Leave me alone. Leave me alone."

Teachers say he doesn't try in school.

Worse with consolation(2); better after being left alone for a while. Doesn't even like his mother to sit close to him when he is upset. He gets up and moves away; as a child, he would run from her. "It's as if he cannot take any more input of any kind."

In grade school, he asked to have his desk turned toward the wall; he didn't want to face the other children.

"I can't do anything right." Becomes frustrated when something doesn't work perfectly (2). Sometimes will break things (2), something he has made, in his rage.

Holds his head(3), with a tormented expression (3), when trying to do schoolwork.

Yet is competent at building and flying intricate remote-control airplanes. His peers in this activity are all adults.

Awkward; drops things (2).

Poor appetite (1); prefers cold drinks (1).

Desires salt (1); likes sweets.

Averse to vegetables (3).

Low energy between 4 and 6 p.m. (2); lies down after school; cannot do homework until 7 or 8 p.m. (2).

Doesn't do chores at home; seems to be because of a tiredness (2), yet will work with his planes endlessly.

During sleep:
- Grinds teeth (2).
- Cries out "mom" or "help" sometimes (2), a shriek as if frightened (3).
- Chewing movements of jaw (2); worse if under stress, such as school pressures.

- Sleeps with eyes half open since a baby (2).
- Sleeps deeply (3); is very hard to awaken, regardless of how long he has slept.

Picks the skin on his fingers while sitting and staring, when he is feeling bad (2); has done this since he was a small child.

Slender face. Asymmetrical: features are smaller on one side. Strained look (1); doesn't look relaxed (no wrinkles or furrows). Looks younger than his age.

Recent mild headaches, which go away spontaneously.

Had a high fever (104°F, 40°C) when five months old; lasted for 48 hours, during which he was totally lethargic, "like a great stupor."

Once, when about two years old, he was dazed and would barely respond after being left with a babysitter. For two or three days, he was drowsy, with eyes dulled and staring blankly. He would respond, but very slowly. The etiology (maybe a fright) was never uncovered.

Was exposed to sewer gas, which was leaking in his house for about two years (1986-1988). He developed chronic respiratory problems, did worse in school, and developed slurred speech, requiring months of speech therapy.

EEG was normal.

Vision and hearing were normal.

Had taken Cicuta (most recent remedy) in 1988, and it seemed to produce some amelioration. (Indications: inattentive; staring while in school.) Previously, had taken Zincum, which definitely helped his symptoms of anxiety, restlessness (especially in the legs), and unrefreshed sleep.

Assessment: Learning problems.

[The speaker asked for suggestions for the prescription. Opium and Helleborus were suggested.]

Case Discussion

Although I had known his mother for years, this was the first time she consulted me about his problem. As I listened to the case, an image began to form in my mind.

Here was a child who had always had difficulty learning in school. My nurse practitioner training automatically prompted me to ask about his vision and hearing. Undoubtedly they had been tested, but I wanted to make sure. Indeed, they were normal. So, he was seeing and hearing well, but could not comprehend.

My mind jumped to one of those few graphic remedy descriptions from the materia medica that seem to remain indelibly engraved in my brain. Hahnemann writes, "a condition where, with sight unimpaired, nothing is seen very fully...; with the hearing perfectly sound, nothing is heard distinctly; with perfectly constituted gustatory organs, everything seems to have lost its taste...."

"What about Helleborus?" I asked. The mother, who is a homeopath, didn't respond, but kept on giving her son's symptoms. She probably thought it was too bizarre a remedy for the case. But, as we talked further, I turned on MacRepertory. I could barely contain my excitement as I scrolled through Roger Morrison's keynotes and Boericke's descriptions of Helleborus.

Then began one of the most joyful experiences of prescribing, when confirmatory questioning elicits strong and definite positive responses! As a result of my questioning, his mother recalled the fever in infancy when he appeared to be in a quiet stupor. She also remembered the episode of unresponsiveness after a probable fright when he was about two years old. She had forgotten these until that moment. Soon she too became interested, and we went through Kent and Clarke, confirming symptoms. It was an incredible learning experience for both of us. I began to feel certain that the remedy would act.

Helleborus niger is made from the tincture of the powdered root of the Christmas rose, otherwise known as snow rose because it blooms from January to March. It is black hellebore because of the color of its root. (White hellebore is Veratrum album; American white hellebore is Veratrum viride.)

This patient's lack of capacity to "see" and "hear" even though his vision and hearing were normal led me to think of Helleborus. I discovered he had many other symptoms of the remedy. There were the two previously mentioned stupor-like states. Helleborus is a "2" in the rubric, "answers slowly." Kent says, "waiting a long time to answer, or not answering at all." This occurs because the mind is not functioning; it is tremendously slowed down.

George Vithoulkas gives the main idea of the Helleborus symptomatology as a kind of stupefaction, an inability to process and perceive the information that the sensory organs transmit to the brain. Vithoulkas says, "Helleborus seems to interrupt communication by stupefying that portion of the brain that receives, processes, and interprets sensory data from the outside world." The sensory organs are intact and functioning, but the *perception* is impaired. The very words used by this patient's mother were, "He hears and sees well, but he just cannot comprehend the instructions."

"Confusion of mind," Kent says, speaking of a delirium, but it is also true for this patient: "He cannot think." It may appear to be a state of dullness or apathy, especially in the earlier stages of the remedy pathology. But often the patient makes a tremendous effort to counter this slowed mind that cannot think. There is a desperation that develops from this inability to comprehend, especially in the later stages of Helleborus. We have the image of our patient, when unable to answer the teacher's questions, holding his head, with a tormented expression on his face, and then running from the room screaming. The experience of the patient is like a living *hell*.

The inability of the mind to function often leads to a tremendous irresolution in Helleborus, but this irresolution was not prominent in this boy.

It is interesting that Helleborus is a "2" in the repertory for "rage." In this case, the patient's rage was caused by his utter frustration at not being able to function in school and to do what was asked of him.

Helleborus is a "2" for "consolation aggravates." Kent describes this in his materia medica.

The generalities in this case are also strong for Helleborus: He is averse to vegetables (Helleborus is a "2"); he has to lie down after school from 4 to 6 p.m.; and he cannot do homework before 8 p.m. Helleborus is a "2" in the rubrics, "worse 4 p.m." and "worse 4 to 8 p.m.," like the more well-known Lycopodium.

There are no strong temperature modalities in Helleborus. This fits with the general lack of perception that is characteristic of this remedy. Kent says, "rarely much disturbed by being touched, or by being covered too warmly, or by not being covered at all. He does not seem to be sensitive to heat or cold...."

Helleborus is a "2" for shrieking during sleep and, likewise, for deep sleep, as we might expect because of the stupor that is characteristic of this remedy. It is also a "2" for grinding the teeth during sleep.

This boy has slept with his eyes half open since he was a baby. Kent, in his description of delirium, mentions that the eyes are partly open. This, in combination with his early stupefying fever, his unresponsiveness after being at the babysitter's, and the presence of his learning disabilities since he began school, suggest that Helleborus might have been indicated quite early in this patient's life.

In school, he did not want to be confronted with extra stimuli. There is an opposite state in Helleborus where, as in the case Clarke cites of a child with seizures followed by a stuporous state, there is a striking amelioration from a strong stimulus, for example a loud noise.

Boericke speaks of the chewing motion of the mouth. Clarke lists "awkwardness" and "dropping things." Kent reads, "...stares at the doctor...with a dazed expression on his face, and picks his finger ends." He is referring to a delirious state, but we have this exact symptom in our patient when he is feeling stressed.

It was on all of these symptoms that I based my prescription of Helleborus.

Plan: Helleborus 10M, one dose.

Follow-Ups: A Remarkable Response to Helleborus

First Follow-Up: December 3, 1989

Doing "unbelievably well."

His mother doesn't have to talk to him about doing his homework.

He is in charge of his life, and happy!

Not failing any of his courses; no criticism from his teachers.

The impetigo-like eruption around his mouth, which he's had chronically off and on, cleared up right after the remedy.

Sleeping well; no teeth grinding or chewing movements since the remedy.

His anxiety is much less; he is more confident; school is not as stressful.

His energy is fine, even after school.

He gets up himself; his mother doesn't have to wake him.

Still has difficulty organizing (2) (i.e., notebook).

No preoccupied look.

No headaches.

Still averse to vegetables (2).

He is having a growth spurt.

This new condition was stable until the last few days, when he contracted a virulent flu that had been going around. Since then:

- Energy dropped (2).
- Chewing movements during sleep (2).
- Two episodes of crying out at night.
- Can't study as well (2).
- Disorganized (2). (Now, he says his ability to organize had improved somewhat between the remedy and the flu.)
- Confidence dropped (2).
- More preoccupied again (1).
- Angry outbursts over trifles (2).

Assessment: Relapse caused by the flu.

Plan: Finals are approaching in school. I planned to repeat the remedy, but his mother waited. He then confessed he had drunk coffee just prior to the relapse and flu. [Editors' Note: Coffee often interferes with the action of homeopathic remedies.]

Second Follow-Up: December 17, 1989

In a few days, he recovered from the flu and from his relapse! (In the past, his flus would linger on.) He is back to where he was before the flu and coffee.

Sleeping well again.

Is having no problems studying; even said he is liking school! ("Biology is very interesting.")

Energy is good.

Averse to milk all his life (1).

His grandmother noticed how clear his speech was and that he spoke with her on the phone for 20 minutes. (Previously, it had been difficult for him to converse for such a long time.)

One rage, but it passed quickly.

A new symptom: If he exerts himself, his face gets hot and itchy (3); it drives him crazy. The same symptom occurs if he gets anxious. (When he had a close call while driving, he had to stop the car because the itching was so bad.)

He is having a growth spurt the past few weeks; needed larger shoes and pants.

Assessment: The patient is better. He has recovered from the flu and relapse (and coffee). The new symptom is most interesting and confirms the remedy! (See the following discussion.)

Plan: Wait.

Third Follow-Up: January 8, 1990

Almost had an accident driving his car. It was a terrible fright (3). His symptoms began to recur right afterwards: couldn't think (2); talking in his sleep (2), and drowsy (2).

Because finals were approaching, his mother gave him another dose of the remedy.

He slept 16 hours the night after the remedy and had an occipital headache for one day. Then he was able to study well for his finals.

Fourth Follow-Up: March 10, 1990

The patient continues to do very well.

Is more independent; socializing a lot with his peers.

Does homework completely on his own (mother no longer needs to nag him).

Getting Bs and Cs in school. Now likes and has improved in science.

His handwriting has changed.

He is more assertive; stands up for his rights. (When a bad storm made him late for school, he convinced the principal to not record this tardiness on his permanent record; previously, he would have simply come home and gone into a rage, screaming and throwing things.)

Sleep is still better: doesn't grind teeth; no chewing movements.

He is not picking his fingers.

Not dropping things.

Sloppy(1). He still could be better organized, but mentally he is much more organized and happy!

"He's really healthy; I don't worry about him anymore, and he used to be my main concern," says his mother.

Assessment: The patient is better.

Plan: Wait.

Fifth Follow-Up: April 9, 1990

The patient continues to do well.

Further Discussion

On follow-up, the patient responded quite well to the remedy. His mental state improved; he began to function well in school. There was no aggravation noted. His energy rose; he was out socializing with his friends instead of lying down between 4 and 8 p.m. The sleep symptoms cleared up. So did the awkwardness and picking of his fingers. His aversion to vegetables decreased slightly.

It is interesting that he relapsed after a bad flu and drinking coffee, and then rallied. Later, a fright caused a relapse. The mother treated the relapse because she was worried about his upcoming final exams. Helleborus is not listed under complaints from fright. However, Vithoulkas has said Helleborus can be useful in symptoms arising from emotional shocks such as fright and grief. It is likely that a fright at the babysitter's resulted in this patient's Helleborus-like state of slowed responsiveness and staring.

An event that confirmed Helleborus to me was the new symptom the patient described in the December 17, 1989, follow-up. He had developed itching and heat on the face that were so intense he had to stop what he was doing. Kent describes a more extreme but, I think, similar state in great detail:

Just imagine these benumbed fingers and hands and limbs, this benumbed skin everywhere. What would be the most natural thing to develop as evidence of the rousing up of this stupid child? (After brain and spinal troubles.) It is necessary for you to know this. It is not really a part of the teaching of the homeopathic materia medica, but you must know what to expect after giving this remedy...Well, that child's fingers will commence to *tingle*. As he comes back to his normal nervous condition, the fingers commence to tingle, the nose and ears tingle, and the child begins to scream and toss back and forth, and roll about the bed. The neighbors will come in and say, "I would send that doctor away unless he gives something to help that child," but just as sure as you do it you will have a dead baby in twenty-four hours. That child is getting well; let him alone.

Kent goes on to advise taking the father aside beforehand and warning him of this reaction and of its necessity to bring about a cure. Then he says not to stay and watch the case too long, or you will be sorely tempted to give a new remedy for this state!

Thus, where there was faulty perception before Helleborus is given, there may be a period after the remedy when sensory perception becomes intensely exaggerated. Kent reassures us, saying it will pass if you give it time. Fortunately, this symptom is now gone in our patient.

So, we see here a case quite nicely covered by Helleborus. The central idea of stupefaction runs through this case from the early history to the lifelong learning disability. Repetition of the remedy after the relapse caused another dramatic amelioration.

I saw another example of Helleborus in an acute case of a one-year-old child with a high fever and pneumonia. He was not originally my patient, so I was not aware of how changed he was from his usual very high-energy state. For four days, I missed the remedy. From the beginning, the parents had said he was "passive," which was unusual for him. Finally, it became clear that there was a 4 to 8 p.m. aggravation of his fever. This led me to prescribe Helleborus, and his pneumonia resolved.

Vithoulkas says that the idea of passiveness pervades Helleborus. Kent reiterates this in comparing Helleborus to the more wild deliriums of Belladonna and Stramonium. Helleborus is useful in other acute states where there is stupefaction; for example, meningitis, severe diarrhea, or severe headaches that stupefy. It is also useful after head injuries when the patient is drowsy and answers very slowly.

Remedies that Compare with Helleborus

Remedies to differentiate from Helleborus include Alumina, Phosphoric acid, Opium, Baryta carbonica, Natrum muriaticum, Staphisagria, Natrum carbonicum, and Zincum.

Alumina has confusion of mind. There is a delayed reaction to stimulation; if you prick an Alumina patient with a pin, the response to pain occurs after a second or two. Cocculus and Plumbum also have this state. Alumina patients may hold or rub their head as they try to think; they also respond slowly to questions. They have severe constipation and impulses or fear from seeing knives, neither of which were present in this patient. They can have a fear of insanity because of their mental confusion, like Helleborus (according to Vithoulkas).

Phosphoric acid is also slow to respond but is more apathetic, with an onset from grief and a desire for juicy things. Vithoulkas says the Helleborus state is not really an apathetic one. Indeed, the emotions are quite alive; it is the mind that is dull.

The stupor of **Opium** is more profound, and its chronic state may be accompanied by sleepiness and constipation. Opium patients are not bothered by their state; Helleborus patients are. In fact, in Opium there is a characteristic anesthesia of parts that should be painful. The Opium state can come on from fright or head injury, as with Helleborus.

Baryta carbonica certainly enters into the differential for this patient with a learning disability. But he does not have a history of tonsillitis and swollen cervical glands, the great shyness, or the aversion to fruit. Baryta carbonica patients tend to bite their nails rather than pick their fingers.

Natrum muriaticum also has the difficulty in learning (repertory: MIND, talk, slow learning to, a "3") and the aggravation from consolation that we see in this patient. But, before giving this remedy, one would like to see more confirmatory symptoms, such as the characteristic aggravation from the sun, desire for salt, aversion to fat, great thirst, sleeping on the left side, claustrophobia, fear of heights, and headaches on waking or worse at 10 a.m. Grief was not mentioned as a major event in this case, although his parents have been separated for many years. Certainly, school has been a source of grief and humiliation for this boy.

Staphisagria is suggested by the humiliation and criticism he has received in school. It can have rage (usually only in the later stages), but again does not cover the case as well as Helleborus. There is no history of styes, excessive masturbation, aggravation from afternoon nap, or desire or aversion to milk to confirm Staphisagria.

Natrum carbonicum has difficulty assimilating on the mental and physical levels and a history of many hurts. But there is no hint in our patient of an aggravation from sun or music, or of the characteristic diarrhea from milk.

Clarke says in his *Relationship of Remedies* that Helleborus is compatible with, and is followed well by, **Zincum**, which had been given in the past to this boy with some amelioration. Zincum is prescribed for overactivity of the nervous system, including twitches or convulsions, and for great restlessness of the legs. In Zincum, the mind is hyperactive.

Conclusion

I had not previously thought of Helleborus for patients with learning problems. It is the most similar remedy for this case, as evidenced by the dramatic change in this boy's life. Our children are our future. It is a tragedy to allow even one child to stumble through life with a "learning disability" when this condition has the possibility to be so successfully treated by homeopathy.

Chipkin: I'm interested to hear any comments and clinical experiences that you want to share.

George Guess: Just one brief comment. Having just read Tutorials in Homeopathy *by Foubister, I want to emphasize what you mentioned in passing. It sounds as if one could interpret this case as an acute effect of a head injury. Foubister was very keen on Helleborus for effects of head injuries, saying it is the major remedy for chronic ill effects of head injuries in children. Foubister cited certain keynotes that are not listed elsewhere, including difficulty in remembering recent events. For those who haven't read the book, I recommend it. One aspect I really liked was the way Foubister would infer that a head injury had occurred and would use that as a confirmation when he suspected a case might need Helleborus. He cited such things as too rapid delivery, difficult delivery, or forceps delivery as possible indications for one of the remedies for head injuries.*

Michael Carlston: Three or four years ago, I gave Helleborus to a patient who had fallen from a 70-foot cliff and was comatose for a couple of weeks. When she came in later for treatment, she was very slow in comprehension and speaking. I gave her the remedy. I knew right away that it was correct because she began speaking so quickly that I had trouble understanding her. Interestingly enough, she also reported the itching that you described in your case. She said all the wounds from the fall itched very intensely for a while after the remedy.

Chipkin: Jennifer, are you going to tell us about your daughter's case?

Jennifer Jacobs: Yes, but first I want to compliment you. That was a great case. I do have an experience using Helleborus. It was several years ago during one of the sessions of the IFH professional course. My husband, Dean Crothers, and my three-year-old daughter were very sick that week with Shigella dysentery. They caught the dysentery from our housekeeper who was from Tonga. Some of her relatives had come to visit and brought along this virulent strain of dysentery from the South Pacific. The housekeeper and I did not catch the dysentery. I don't know what that says about our vital force, whether it's high or low.

Anyway, my daughter was lying on the sofa. We had to put disposable diapers underneath her because the stool would come out involuntarily in bloody, jelly-like clumps. I was giving her Mercury and the more usual diarrhea and dysentery remedies, but nothing was happening. I was getting concerned because she became quite unresponsive. She was just lying there in a daze.

Finally, she got to the point where she started picking her lips. It was a delirium-like state, where she was unconsciously picking the skin off her lips. So I rushed to the repertory and looked under that symptom. Helleborus was listed. I found it was also listed for the jelly-like stool. I gave it to her, and the case turned around immediately.

Chipkin: I recall from the notes on your daughter's case that she would open her mouth to talk, move her lips, but not quite get the words out. Was that part of the stupor?

Jennifer Jacobs: Yes.

Jody Shevins: I had a classic Helleborus case. A little girl injured her head and then all her schoolwork fell apart. She was in a stupor-like state. At the point of the impact of the injury, she developed a bald spot even though the skin didn't break. As soon as she took the remedy, her memory and mental functioning came back. She brightened up, and all her hair grew back. One of the little keynotes in Helleborus is that they will lose their hair and nails.

Chipkin: Interesting. Anybody else who has prescribed Helleborus?

Steve Olson: I recently had a case of a woman who wanted to commit suicide. She sighed a lot. I gave her Helleborus and she is doing well.

Chipkin: Did she also have anxiety and anguish about not being able to function mentally?

Steve Olson: Yes, it was tremendous. She couldn't think. She said that her husband couldn't even have normal conversations with her anymore because she really couldn't think.

Chipkin: Yes, that symptom can certainly lead the Helleborus patient to become suicidal.

Edward Chapman, MD

A CASE
OF
NARCOLEPSY

Edward Chapman, MD, is a board-certified family physician with specialization in the use of homeopathic methods. He received his BS from the University of New Hampshire and an MD from George Washington University in 1979. After completing a three-year Family Practice residency at Brown University, he apprenticed in homeopathy for one year with David Wember, MD, and Catherine Coulter, MA, in Washington, D.C. His practice is in classical homeopathy and family medicine in Newton, Massachusetts, with hospital privileges at Mt. Auburn, Newton-Wellesley, and Malden Hospitals.

Ted is president-elect of the American Institute of Homeopathy. He is involved in medical research and education, and is conducting a study of the homeopathic treatment of premenstrual syndrome. He is also a clinical instructor at Harvard Medical School in the "Patient/Doctor" course for first-year medical students. Other physicians and medical students regularly sit in with him and his patients to learn homeopathy.

Description of the Patient

The patient was a 30-year-old Norwegian woman, born on June 21, 1959. She was single, working in sales in Boston, and going to school in fashion design.

Appearance: She was very tall and thin (5'10"; 129 lbs), with full lips, a pasty, pale complexion like one who never sees the sun, dark shaggy hair, and blue eyes. She was very soft-spoken; her voice was relatively monotonic. Her demeanor was depressed and droopy, but she lit up when she smiled. Her physical exam was otherwise unremarkable.

Chief Complaint: Narcolepsy for the past three years. Current medication: Ritalin 5 mg, six per day.

Patient History:

Date	Age	Event	Consequence
1959		Born in Norway	
1965	15	Mother: psychiatric hospitalization	Depressed; "I couldn't help my mother."

Date	Age	Event	Consequence
1980	21	Immigrated to U.S. for school and travel	
1981	22	Married a U.S. citizen	
1983	23	Divorced	
1984	24	Graduated from the university; returned to Norway	
1986	26	Onset of narcolepsy	
1987	27	Began therapy; started Ritalin	Depressed; moved back to U.S.
1988	28	Acupressure	Phobias were better; symptoms improved; cataplexy was better

Family History:
- General comments: "Dysfunctional; too strict." Three younger sisters.
- Mother: Coronary artery disease; mental health problems.
- Aunt: Leukemia.
- Father: Cerebral vascular disease; arthritis.
- Paternal grandmother: Stomach cancer.
- Sister No. 3: Anorexia.

A Freezing of Emotional Expression

Initial Interview: August 4, 1989

The narcolepsy began in 1986 while she was in Norway. She had returned to Norway from the United States after finishing her B.A. at the University of Minnesota in 1984. The initial symptoms were visions on awakening of people and shapes that moved. They frightened her and made her feel as if she were going insane. She discovered that if she felt angry at them, she could get them to go away.

Excessive sleepiness began about the same time. Before this symptom began to occur, she described herself as a night owl. She would go to bed at 2 a.m., often experience initial difficulty getting to sleep, and feel sluggish when she woke in the morning. Since the narcolepsy began, she could fall asleep any time, often inappropriately without warning while talking, reading, on the subway, and at work. Her nighttime sleep also became different, "lighter, full of vivid, frightening dreams so real that it feels like a different reality."

In addition to the visions and sleep disturbances, she noted two other symptoms. On waking at night she would find it impossible to move, "like I'm lying under an iron blanket." If she felt any strong emotion or upset, such as anger, crying, or laughter, she would "fall over with sudden weakness." As a result, she said, "I want to stay neutral."

It took her two years to be diagnosed as narcoleptic. The diagnosis was associated with the classic tetrad: hypersomnia (100 percent of the cases), cataplexy (sudden onset of muscle weakness with emotion, 70 percent of the cases), sleep paralysis (unable to move on waking, 50 percent of the cases), and hypnagogic hallucinations (vivid illusions either during sleep or during the period of paralysis, 25 percent of the cases). The natural history of narcolepsy usually shows an onset of symptoms in early adulthood, persisting throughout the adult period, and possibly decreasing in frequency in old age.

She left Norway and returned to the United States a few months after the onset of symptoms in 1986, because she couldn't work and the darkness aggravated her overall state. She went into therapy in 1987 because she felt depressed and had begun to experience phobias. These phobias included a feeling of "someone behind me or in the next room," a fear of crowds, and an anxiety about her appearance typified by the fear that her odor was offensive or that her menses would appear and show. These fears were somewhat diminished by the therapy, but she continued to be self-conscious and to have only a small handful of friends, feeling embarrassed to be emotional with people.

She rarely cried, but tended to brood on feelings. She only recently discovered anger, sadness, and jealousy as emotions, and remarked that "they solve many problems." She rarely expressed anger. When asked about anger, she replied, "This illness has taken away my physical strength." She was learning to say "no." She had recently discontinued therapy. She feared support groups for narcoleptics. "I don't want to know how bad it can be; I've gotten better because I continued to fight. I don't want to be burdened by others' troubles. It takes all my energy to live for myself." She fears work discrimination because of her illness.

She had done some acupressure, which helped the cataplexy symptoms somewhat; she now only collapsed when she laughed. To control the sleepiness, she was relying on Ritalin, taking six to eight 5-mg tablets per day.

The sleepiness was worse before and during menses, if she had a respiratory illness, and after eating. Other premenstrual symptoms included irritability; abdominal bloating; cravings for salt, grease (normally averse to fat), chips, and chocolate; sore breasts, which would increase by one size before the menses; and acne on the face (also aggravated by humidity and chemicals).

Other symptoms included weakness of the left knee, with pain when bearing weight; tense muscles in the neck; achiness of her joints; a tendency for the eyes to cross if tired; sensitive scalp with white, dry dandruff in the winter; a tendency to sinusitis with colds; a dry mouth ("I try to drink but it dries out faster than I'm able to drink"); frequent vaginal yeast infections (allergies to Flagyl and tetracycline); and sensitive stomach with frequent painless, loose stools when feeling anxious. She smoked cigarettes, one pack per day, and experienced some shortness of breath when running.

She was chilly, hated the cold weather, and liked the sun, although it made her feel tired. She felt tired on waking, was awake by 10 a.m., and got sluggish after lunch. She slept on her side, curled up and covered.

No laboratory studies were performed.

Discussion of Possible Remedies

Chapman: Would anyone like to suggest a prescription?

Durr Elmore: Nux moschata, because of the sleepiness and the dryness, the very dry mouth. I didn't repertorize it much. The remedy just came to mind, but it was clearly indicated for the symptoms I did look up, such as the dry mouth. Probably Nux moschata is the primary remedy for narcolepsy.

Chapman: Anybody else? Somebody just said Opium. Does anybody want to defend Opium as a prescription?

Rick Wilkinson: I was the one who said Opium. It just struck me that some of the characteristics that you mentioned, such as the lack of energy and any vital reaction, indicate that the patient doesn't have much of anything coming out. It's almost a deadness while she is talking to you. And besides that, Opium has the dry mouth.

Tom Kruzel: Nux moschata sounds pretty good. We also noted when looking through the repertory that there are a number of symptoms of Nux vomica as well, including the delusion of having the person beside them.

Bill Shevin: There are symptoms of Medorrhinum, of course, and also you could look at the foods and think of Carcinosin, especially with the sore breasts. Medorrhinum came out initially, but I'm not sure it covers the sleep situation very well.

Chapman: Well, I basically saw the case the same way that Dr. Elmore sees it. It couldn't really be anything else. Let me explain my analysis in more detail.

Evaluation of Initial Interview

The center of the pathology of this case was in the nervous system: sleepiness, cataplexy, and sleep paralysis. Etiologic factors included losses and disappointments leading to repression of feelings in adolescence or earlier. The striking aspect of the emotional life was the lack of awareness of emotions. Rather than repression, the picture was more of a freezing of expression on the emotional plane: "I'm just discovering emotions." The effect of emotional expression within the pathology was collapse (cataplexy); when the underlying emotions would find expression (hallucinations on waking), it would lead to paralysis.

Based on the repertorization of the selected rubrics and on analysis of the case, the primary remedies considered were Nux moschata and Natrum muriaticum. The background of the case, from the childhood and basic emotionality, strongly suggests a Natrum muriaticum constitution. However, the peculiarity and intensity of the sleep symptoms lead one to consider a remedy with these particular characteristics. Nux moschata fills that bill with its overpowering sleepiness, fogginess of mind, and dryness. The patient was dependent on Ritalin to function, and therefore it was unlikely that a single dose of the remedy would hold.

Plan: Nux moschata 200c (Boiron-Borneman) was prescribed. A vial of 30c was provided in the event that the single-dose technique did not hold.

The Patient "Wakes Up"

First Follow-Up: September 1, 1989

The patient took an initial dose of the remedy and was better. Something was released; she felt more control over the sleepiness and other symptoms. The improvement lasted for two to three days. After speaking with me, she went on a daily dose of the 30c potency of the remedy.

Better all over; less nervous; more confident.

More sensitive and emotional; not holding back, ignoring, or hiding feelings.

Crying more easily (2).

More depressed, "fighting an old feeling."

Bad dreams. Waking feeling as if something bad has happened. "Like I've woken up, wondering who I am, what's happening in my life. The illness has been like a death. I've given up so much."

Sleepiness was not much different, but using only one to two Ritalin per day. Especially tired 1 to 3 p.m. Wakes in the morning feeling tired.

Mouth is less dry.

Menses are lighter; fewer cramps; no PMS; breasts are less sore.

Acne is worse.

Fewer cravings.

More comfortable in crowds.

Smoking less.

Assessment: The remedy clearly acted in a curative direction and with it came a clarity of the patient's experience of her condition. The intriguing aspect of this interview was how it clarified the symptoms of the case. The dullness of mind seemingly affected the clarity of the expression of the case at the initial interview.

"It's like I've woken up." The difference between the interviews highlights how, as homeopaths, we must often infer symptoms from behaviors. The understanding of the remedy image is an evolving process. **The pathology of Nux moschata involves a falling asleep of the patient to herself.** This may make it a difficult remedy to identify when the physical pathology is not highly evolved.

Plan: Nux moschata 30c was continued daily.

Second Follow-Up: October 11, 1989

More energetic; socializing more.

Excited about the changes; aware how precious time is.

Feeling that, as an oldest child, she was taken for granted. Now, doesn't want the responsibility.

Using one Ritalin per day.

Menses are less painful.

Fewer food cravings.

More acne.

Assessment: The patient's understanding of herself was continuing to evolve, going back to basic childhood adaptations.

Plan: Nux moschata 30c, daily. I suggested that she might try to stop the remedy.

A Relapse After Discontinuing the Remedy

Third Follow-Up: November 12, 1989

Stopped the remedy; felt insecure and tired.

Started the remedy again.

Allergy symptoms: nose stuffed; eyes irritated; better with cold applications; aggravated by make-up.

Generally felt up and down. Physically felt drained more easily.

Felt lonely, homesick, and resigned.

Anxiety attacks; felt frozen. "There's something wrong with me. I'm strange, limited. People are laughing at me. I'm marked, like my period is running through."

Aversion to company.

Skin is clearing up.

Menstrual cramps are more painful and prolonged.

Sleepy after lunch.

Ritalin, once a day.

Assessment: The patient experienced a relapse of the symptoms on discontinuing the remedy. New symptoms of the allergy were developing. Could this be a proving? Older emotions, such as panic and loneliness, were arising in a mild form. The acne was clearing. Either this represented a continued improvement or a movement of the pathology back toward the core. With the general deterioration, the latter seemed more likely.

Plan: Nux moschata 200c, three doses, 12 hours apart. Continue 30c as needed. The 30c potency was probably no longer active and would act as a placebo or would, if active, continue to prove itself in the patient.

A Remedy for Acute Symptoms

Fourth Follow-Up: December 7, 1989

Acute symptoms; cold symptoms. Severe sore throat, better with warm drinks. When swallows, tends to choke; goes down the wrong way. Worse on the left side. Ears congested. Hot and cold. Cough, as if from dust.

Sleepiness is a lot better. Hasn't needed Ritalin since a few days after taking the 200c of Nux moschata.

Anxiety is a bit better.

Just before getting sick was "Looking at myself. It came in waves. Realized low self-confidence. Don't believe in myself. Settle for less than I deserve. People use me."

Stools are loose (an old symptom).

Anxiety is worse in the morning, on rising.

Desires seaweed, salty chips(2), and soya milk(2).

Objective: Right ear was red; good movement of the ear drum. Pharynx was red, and lungs were clear.

Assessment: The acute symptoms clearly indicated Arsenicum album. The intensity of the symptoms made treatment necessary. The deeper constitutional case continued to evolve in a curative direction.

Plan: Arsenicum album 30c, every three to four hours as needed. Nux moschata 200c, to hold.

Fifth Follow-Up: January 11, 1990

On the verge of needing Ritalin, but not using it. The 30c of Nux moschata was not holding. Has used the 200c of Nux moschata several times.

Skin is dry and breaking out on her legs; round, red, itching (like when she was 14 and 15 years old).

Wanting to be more social.

Notices mind goes blank (to sleep) momentarily, at which time she feels paranoid.

Many feelings arose after the cold; so many things and too much to handle that fast.

Dreams are less vivid.

Menses: bleeds for one week.

Assessment: The old symptoms continued to appear on the surface. There was a deepening understanding of her own emotions; she was experiencing them consciously and therefore less in her dream life. Sleep symptoms were on the verge of relapsing.

Plan: Nux moschata 1M.

Another Remedy Layer is Presented

Sixth Follow-Up: February 28, 1990

Used the remedy daily in 30c potency and twice in the 1M, after which she gets sleepier for two to three days and is then much better. Used Ritalin once in six weeks. Needing to nap less after work, although is a bit sleepy from 3 to 6 p.m.

Feels a need to be with people:

I've been asleep so long. I'm curious about people. It's easier to be with them. There's so much to catch up with. It is hard to keep pace. There are so many things I want to have. Anger is coming up at my parents. My mother was always busy. I was kept back, not allowed to have friends. I was my father's princess; then, when I went through puberty, he was constantly an authority, saying "no."

Skin is better.

Mouth is dry, if nervous and talking.

Less chilly.

Stomach and bowels are so-so.

Menses: flow less heavy; no breast tenderness.

Craving salt, chocolate (2), and sweets before menses.

Assessment: She was experiencing a new sense of confidence and desire for intimacy. The anger at her parents was beginning to raise its head. There was an increase in her craving for salt. A Natrum muriaticum layer seemed to be presenting itself.

Plan: Nux moschata 30c; 1M to hold.

Seventh Follow-Up: March 24, 1990

I saw the patient on an emergency basis. She called on a Saturday, saying she "couldn't stand it any more."

Severe neck pain with numbness for two weeks, extending to the occiput, shoulders, and right arm. Turning the head was almost impossible.

"Spoke to my sister who is very depressed and won't help herself. I can't let go. I feel helpless, like when I was 15. I couldn't help her (mother was hospitalized with depression). I'm terribly angry at my sister for not helping herself."

Observation: Marked tension in the right trapezius, with 45-degree rotation. Neurological examination was normal.

Assessment: The Natrum muriaticum picture had presented itself in an acute cervical neck spasm, the intensity of which made treatment necessary. The trigger factor for this state was the family crisis, from which she struggled to maintain her independence although living across the Atlantic.

Plan: Cervical collar. Natrum muriaticum 200c, every 12 hours for three doses. Stop Nux moschata.

No Ritalin for Over Two Months

Eighth Follow-Up: April 18, 1990

Her neck was significantly better after two to three days. Used the collar on and off for a week.

Developed a severe headache one week later, which resolved itself in several days.

Felt much better emotionally over this period.

I reviewed the state of the narcolepsy:

She was not using any Nux moschata and had not taken any Ritalin for 2 1/2 months.

She was sleepy only after eating, hardly a problem. She still had weakness of the legs, was surprised when she was tired, and said the cataplexy was 60 percent better since beginning homeopathy (seven months).

Her voice also was affected by laughing, during which she experienced a tension in the larynx.

Sleep paralysis occurred rarely when waking from naps.

Occasionally her sleep was very light, when she heard voices and had a "threatened feeling, like someone is there." One of her first memories was a nightmare that recurred in childhood, she was "trapped and couldn't get out, not able to move." She would wake up and cry.

After this discussion, she brought up, somewhat embarrassedly, a concern over how hard it was for her to climax in sex. "Sex is frustrating. I get up there, then something says 'no,' a fear of letting go, losing control." She was very concerned about this, although she was not in an active relationship. Since taking Nux moschata, orgasms have been easier, she's more sensitive to touch, and has been crying more easily at movies.

Assessment: New information came up, which raised concern over the possibility of sexual abuse. I mentioned this to her, and she stated that she had wondered about it but didn't have memories. Her previous psychiatrist had raised the issue.

Plan: No prescription.

Sheryl Kipnis: Two questions. First, in October when she was doing so much better, why did you discontinue the homeopathic remedy instead of discontinuing the Ritalin when she was just down to one pill a day?

Chapman: I really didn't discontinue the remedy. I told her to see if she needed to take it every day, and she said that she felt worse when she didn't take it daily. Shortly after that, in late November, she dropped the Ritalin.

Sheryl Kipnis: Earlier in the day a comment was made that we homeopaths are always experimenting with potency and repetition of dose. So my second question, and I am sure you were expecting it, is whether you had any particular rationale in continuing the 30c daily dosage and then giving her occasional doses of higher potencies or if you were just experimenting.

Chapman: Well, it was partly an experiment. I felt that as long as she was using the Ritalin it probably was not going to hurt. I guess I'm not really comfortable repeating the 200c dosage every day. So, I had her continue what she was doing, and my impression is that the occasional doses of a higher potency may have moved the case to the next stage. I'm certainly not an expert in these matters. But in this case it worked fine and didn't cause any problems. That much is clear from the case itself.

Summary

This case to date has two layers, and a third begins to raise its head as a possibility. The first layer, the narcoleptic pattern, was covered by Nux moschata. The second layer, the underlying emotional suppression, was addressed by Natrum muriaticum. A third layer is suggested by the possibility of sexual abuse.

This case is special to me because, as the patient's understanding of her condition unfolds, my awareness of the remedy image as it is expressed in this patient also unfolds. As I heard a famous homeopath once say, "Our patients are our best teachers."

George Guess, MD, DHt

A CASE OF
PRIMARY
HYPOTHYROIDISM

George Guess, MD, DHt, is in private practice in Asheville, North Carolina. He is a graduate of the Medical College of Virginia, Richmond, and completed his Family Medicine residency at Southern Illinois University. George was a graduate of the first IFH Professional Course (taught by Bill Gray) in 1978. In subsequent years, he has studied extensively with George Vithoulkas and, in 1984, spent one year at the Athenian Center for Homeopathic Medicine in Greece, where he was awarded the Diploma of the Athenian School of Homeopathic Medicine. He is a past member of the NCH Board of Directors and is currently chairman of the AIH Legal Committee and president of the American Board of Homeotherapeutics. George is also involved in the ongoing transcription and editing of Vithoulkas' Living Materia Medica.

A Diffusely Enlarged Thyroid

Initial Visit: April 5, 1988

A 30-year-old woman, recently a mother (seven months ago), presented with the complaint of hypothyroidism. In March, her thyroid values were as follows: T4 = 1.0 (normal range is 4.5-13.0) and TSH = 50 (normal range is 0.4-6.0).

She complained of the following:

No energy (3) for 2 1/2 months, worse in the morning on waking (2) and from 5 to 9 p.m. (1).

Roughness in the throat (1).

Goiter.

Poor appetite, without weight loss.

Soreness of muscles in the shoulders (trapezia; worse reaching up), back, and legs (1).

For the past three months, her extremities have often fallen asleep; the arm and hand on the side lain on would go numb; the leg crossed over the other becomes numb.

Tired (sleepy) but on lying down at night to sleep she becomes anxious and wakeful; feels restless (3) and wiggles her legs (2). She then feels that she should be doing something, should go somewhere (2). She is anxious and restless when lying down during the day (2). Her legs are also restless when sitting (2).

There is much inertia to overcome before she can start working at home (2). She has a mellow temperament; not easily upset; no fears. Often feels she should be doing something; likes to be active. She is sympathetic (1), confident, assertive, and social. She used to be anxious before tests (2).

Sexual sphere is normal.

Desires ice cream (3) (all her life) and sweets (2) (more recently).

Averse to spicy food (2).

Was very thirsty; now is thirstless (2).

Appetite is normal.

She is exhausted for one hour after waking in the morning and is averse to getting out of bed then (3).

Averse to excess heat (1). Is all right in the sun. She always has very cold hands and feet (3), and is worse in cold air. Sensitive to cold drafts (1). Little perspiration.

Dry skin, mostly on the hands (2), with some cracking of the skin on the fingertips (1). Her nails flake and chip (1).

After having had no dental cavities in the preceding 10 years, she recently had several cavities.

Some dizziness when she is tired and in the early evening.

Physical Examination: The patient is moderately obese and fair-skinned. The exam was unremarkable except for a diffusely enlarged, firm thyroid.

> *Guess: That's the case as it originally presented itself. Do you have any suggestions for remedies?*

Sheryl Kipnis: I have an idea. I was struck by two symptoms in the case. One is the great fatigue and the other is the restlessness. They seem contradictory. The other symptom that stood out for me was the difficulty she is having with her nails and her teeth, which seems to be associated with the hypothyroid problem. This makes me think about Calcarea carbonica, calcium metabolism. The sluggishness makes me think about a Calcarea remedy, but the restlessness, the goiter, and the enlargement of the glands make me think about Iodium. This raises the possibility of Calcarea iodata, but I have no experience with the remedy. Boericke does mention thyroid enlargement and cracking of the skin for Calcarea iodata. The patient noticed both of these symptoms.

Guess: That's a great idea. Anybody else?

Audience: I guess I will suggest the obvious. There are some confirmatories for Zincum metallicum, but I don't know that much about the remedy in this context. The repertory lists it under "swelling of the external throat," although it is not under "goiter." This remedy obviously has the restlessness, the cracking of the skin, the teeth falling out, and the energy worse in the evening. So I'll suggest Zincum metallicum.

Jeff Baker: I agree with Dr. Kipnis. I think the case has a look of Calcarea, but I'm thinking of Calcarea sulphurica. It seems to run through the case fairly well. The anxiety while lying is a relatively small rubric but is quite characteristic of the case. Calcarea sulphurica is one of only nine remedies listed in that rubric. I think the remedy should be there, actually. Also, the remedy is worse in cold drafts. The food cravings have both a Calcarea and a Sulphur look to them. In the repertory, Calcarea sulphurica is a goiter remedy in italics.

Guess: Thanks. That's another great thought.

Audience: I have a thought too, which is also along the Calcarea line. But I would recommend Rhus toxicodendron, because here is a woman who is very fatigued and is very restless. She feels that she has to be doing something all the time. The main symptom for me in this case is the restlessness while lying down and the restlessness in the legs. She is also worse from cold air and drafts. If you look at the case you think, "Maybe this woman is Calcarea carbonica." But Rhus toxicodendron seems to cover this case. Maybe she needs Rhus toxicodendron now and Calcarea carbonica later.

Guess: The remedy that cured her is often confused with Rhus toxicodendron. But, initially, I did not prescribe the correct remedy. I first gave her Calcarea carbonica, with no effect. Let's look at a more detailed analysis of the case.

Case Analysis and Differential Discussion

I chose the following symptoms for repertorization:

1.	SLEEP:	Unrefreshing
2.	MIND:	Restlessness, evening, bed in
3.	MIND:	Anxiety, evening, bed in
4.	MIND:	Restlessness, lying, while
5.	SLEEP:	Sleeplessness, evening, bed, after going to
6.	STOMACH:	Desires, sweets
7.	STOMACH:	Desires, ice cream
8.	STOMACH:	Thirstless
9.	EXTREMITIES:	Restlessness, sitting, while
10.	MIND:	Indolence
11.	TEETH:	Caries, decayed, hollow
12.	EXTREMITIES:	Dryness, hands
13.	EXTREMITIES:	Cracked skin, hands
14.	EXTERNAL THROAT:	Goiter

The repertorizations, using MacRepertory's Complete Repertory, revealed the following:

4/88 – Totality

	Phos.	Lyc.	Calc.	Puls.	Sulph.	Mag-m.	Sep.	Kali-c.	Nat-m.	Ars.	Hep.	Nux-v.
Total	22	20	19	18	17	16	16	15	15	14	14	14
Rubrics	12	9	8	8	8	8	8	8	8	7	9	8
Sleep; UNREFRESHING												
Mind; RESTLESSNESS; evening; bed, in												
Mind; ANXIETY; evening; bed, in												
Mind; RESTLESSNESS; lying, while												
Sleep; SLEEPLESSNESS; evening; bed,...												
Stomach; DESIRES; sweets												
Stomach; DESIRES; ice cream												
Stomach; THIRSTLESS												
Extremities; RESTLESSNESS; sitting,...												
Mind; INDOLENCE												
Teeth; CARIES, decayed, hollow												
Extremities; DRYNESS; Hands												
Extremities; CRACKED skin; Fingers												
External Throat; GOITRE												

4/88 – totality; strange, rare, peculiar; small remedies; keynotes

	Calc.	Mag-m.	Ambr.	Am-c.	Mag-c.	Nat-c.	Bar-c.	Ph-ac.	Nit-ac.	Petr.	Sabad.	Tub.
Total	19	16	13	12	12	13	12	13	12	9	10	10
Rubrics	8	8	7	8	8	8	7	6	6	6	6	6
Sleep; UNREFRESHING	■	■	▦	■	■	▦	▦	▦	■	▦	▦	■
Mind; RESTLESSNESS; evening; bed, in		■		▦								
Mind; ANXIETY; evening; bed, in	▦	▦	■	▦	▦	▦	▦		▦			
Mind; RESTLESSNESS; lying, while		▦										
Sleep; SLEEPLESSNESS; evening; bed,...		▦	■		▦				▦			
Stomach; DESIRES; sweets	▦	▦		■	▦	■	▦		▦		▦	▦
Stomach; DESIRES; ice cream	■											▦
Stomach; THIRSTLESS			▦	▦	▦	▦	▦		■	▦		▦
Extremities; RESTLESSNESS; sitting,...		▦										
Mind; INDOLENCE	▦	▦	▦	▦	▦	▦	▦	▦	■	▦	▦	▦
Teeth; CARIES, decayed, hollow	▦	▦	▦	▦	▦	▦	▦	▦	▦	▦	▦	▦
Extremities; DRYNESS; Hands					▦	■	▦				▦	
Extremities; CRACKED skin; Fingers	■				▦		▦		▦		■	
External Throat; GOITRE	■		▦	■	■	▦						▦

It is apparent from the results of the repertorization that the following remedies merit our consideration: Calcarea carbonica, Lycopodium, Phosphorus, Ammonium carbonicum, Magnesia carbonica, and Magnesia muriatica. Which of these seems to best fit this case?

Calcarea carbonica is certainly a major goiter remedy, and its overall symptom profile closely mimics the hypothyroid state. In this case, many of the patient's symptoms are shared with Calcarea carbonica: indolence, lethargy, desire for ice cream and sweets, cold hands and feet, soreness from exertion, obesity, dental caries, anxiety in the evening in bed, dry and cracked skin of the hands, and rough throat. There are no absolute contraindications for Calcarea carbonica, except for its failure to cover the strongest and most peculiar aspects of this case.

Lycopodium repertorizes quite well, as you will note, and it figures prominently in the repertory for anxiety and restlessness in the evening in bed; the pretest anxiety also matches Lycopodium. Certain confirmatory symptoms are present: desiring sweets and feeling unrefreshed in the morning. The aggravation between 5 and 9 p.m. is only minimal in this case and, consequently, not a confirmation. We lack the characteristic gastrointestinal symptoms, sleeping on the right side, and other symptoms. But, most importantly, as with Calcarea carbonica, Lycopodium does not best cover the most striking symptoms of this case.

Phosphorus is contraindicated by the strong thirstlessness, and, other than the strong desire for ice cream, there are no confirming symptoms for this remedy.

Ammonium carbonicum has an image that is not consistent with this case. It is more appropriate for heart or lung (and menstrual) pathology. We don't have the characteristic dyspnea or obstructed respiration in sleep, the aggravation at 3 a.m., the acrid discharges, and other such symptoms.

Magnesia carbonica is a thought, but not a good one. It is a goiter remedy. On repertorization, it covers some of the case, especially the unrefreshing sleep, as is characteristic of the Magnesias. However, there is one symptom in this case that flies in the face of Magnesia carbonica: the anxiety that arises on lying down in bed at night. According to George Vithoulkas and J.H. Clarke, the anxiety and foreboding that something will happen evaporates upon going to bed in the Magnesia carbonica patient. Further, in this case, the image of Magnesia carbonica is lacking: the weak, debilitated state with anxiety and liver disturbance or neuralgias, or menstrual complaints.

Finally, we come to **Magnesia muriatica**. The most striking aspect of this case is the anxiety, restlessness, and sleeplessness that arise immediately on lying down in the evening to go to sleep. This symptom cannot be explained by hypothyroidism. This symptom, as you know, is a grand keynote of Magnesia muriatica. In addition, some of the other symptoms of the case are covered by Magnesia muriatica, as a glance at a materia medica will reveal: desire for sweets, indolence, dental caries, rough throat, and, more importantly, unrefreshed sleep — a keynote of this remedy. The fact that it is not a "goiter remedy" must be ignored, although, as you will see, I initially failed on that count. We might also extrapolate from the presence of Magnesia carbonica in the goiter rubric that other Magnesias might also be useful for this pathology.

Certainly, there is not a lot of similarity between this case and the classic description of the symptomatology of Magnesia muriatica. But the common symptoms do share similarity to a degree: worse from the cold; repugnance to exertion; dry, rough throat; pain as from a bruise in the small of the back; numbness of the arms; drawing in the shoulder joint; heaviness and aching of the legs; uneasiness and tension of the thighs; and unrefreshing sleep — tired in the morning (Clarke).

The case becomes strikingly similar, however, when we read Kent's description of one aspect of this remedy:

> Restlessness, fidgetiness throughout the body, coupled with anxiety. This comes on at any time, but it is worse at night in bed and still worse on closing the eyes to go to sleep. When he closes the eyes, he becomes so anxious, restless and fidgety that he must throw the covers off, take a long breath or do something. He is kept awake at night by the anxious feeling.

Of course, Magnesia muriatica is best known as a remedy for impaired digestion and liver dysfunction; however, as Vithoulkas has noted, it may be appropriate for any condition when anxiety and restlessness on lying in bed (and closing the eyes) figure prominently.

The theme of duty and of feeling overloaded with tasks and responsibilities, which Vithoulkas has identified as being characteristic of Magnesia muriatica, is touched upon in this case. Note her comment that when she feels restless and anxious on lying down at night, she "feels...that she should be doing something, should go somewhere." Also, she comments that in general she often feels she should be doing something. Compare this with Vithoulkas' statements:

> They are anxious to accomplish goals or fulfill promises. They become anxious if they cannot accomplish these goals, so anxious that they cannot sleep. Their frustrated sense of duty (and their sensitivity to others, with regard to injustices perpetrated) causes them to become restless and fidgety. In fact, one of the possible causations of the Magnesia muriatica pathology is their inability to accomplish tasks. As a result of their fitful sleep (and especially when the liver is dysfunctional) they awaken in the morning feeling totally unrefreshed.

Plan: The above considerations, conducted at leisure after the patient's visit, did not adequately impose themselves upon my mind during the interview. Consequently, Calcarea carbonica 10M was prescribed.

Results of the Calcarea Carbonica Prescription

May 11, 1988

T4 = 0.7

The patient was very tired (3). No other changes in symptomatology.

Assessment: There was no apparent action from Calcarea carbonica, and her T4 is even lower. Another remedy is required.

Plan: After further study, Magnesia muriatica 200c was prescribed.

Results of the Magnesia Muriatica Prescription

June 23, 1988

Feels "okay."

Energy is still low, perhaps slightly better.

Still feels tight in the throat in the morning; raspy voice in the morning; a bad taste in the mouth then too (2). "Lump in the throat (3)." Dysphagia in the morning (2) due to a tight, dry sensation.

Anxious restlessness at night is much better; there is also no restlessness now on lying down during the day, as there had been before.

No muscle soreness.

Slight tendency for extremities to go to sleep.

Wakens in the morning feeling generally okay, unless a rough day before.

Less leg restlessness when sitting.

Energy is low between 1 and 4 p.m. (2).

Not chilly, but doesn't feel the heat of this hot summer.

Low thirst (2).

Desires sweets (1), salty, ice cream (2), and breads (1).

Averse to spicy (2).

Hair falls out. Dry scalp.

Nails and hands are better.

Moderate appetite. Has lost weight, approximately seven or eight pounds.

Assessment: Now we can see definite signs of positive change. Most notably, the morning energy is markedly better, muscle soreness is gone, overall energy is slightly improved, and there is a significant weight loss. Especially noteworthy now is the absence of nocturnal restlessness. Although there are persisting throat complaints and a continuing low energy, I would be loathe to represcribe Magnesia muriatica now that the keynote of nocturnal restlessness on lying down is gone.

The next remedy is not clear. I considered remedies with throat constriction from goiter, such as Calcarea sulphurica, Lycopodium, Spongia, and Crotalus cascavella.

Plan: Measure T4. The result, T4 = 4.0, suggests that the wisest course is no remedy at this time!

The Magnesia Muriatica is Repeated

July 25, 1988

Her weight continues to slowly decrease.

Throat has been raspy and dry (2) for the past four days; before then, she suffered no throat symptoms at all.

Energy is a little better; it is worse on rainy days (2). Afternoon slump is not as bad.

For the past two weeks has been having trouble falling asleep (2) due to anxiety; is not restless. This is worse on the days she is tired. Some nightmares. Trouble waking in the morning (2).

Less sensitive to cold. No cold, numb limbs. Less dryness of hair. Nails and hands are better. Some hair loss.

Clumsy with hands (1).

Thirst is slightly increased.

Desires sweets (1), bread and cereals (2), and ice cream (2).

Averse to spicy foods.

Assessment: She is still better since the original prescription of Magnesia muriatica. Interestingly, the throat symptoms subsided without another remedy. The slow pace of recovery and the return of Magnesia muriatica symptoms, namely the morning aggravation and anxious wakefulness at night, suggest the appropriateness of repeating Magnesia muriatica.

Plan: Magnesia muriatica 200c.

Continued Improvement and the Remedy Image Changes

August 29, 1988

Her energy is better.

For the past week and a half she has been wide awake the minute she hits the bed, experiencing many thoughts at that time about what she has to do the next day (3). Not restless. Also awakens about every hour (2). Sleeps on her back. Tired in the afternoon (2:30 to 3 p.m.) (1). Okay on waking now.

Sore, bruised angle of right jaw for two weeks; worse when opening the mouth (2).

Slightly dry throat.

No restless legs.

No hand clumsiness.

Weight continues to fall, for a total loss of 14 pounds.

Sex is okay.

Wandering thoughts when concentrating (2). Some trouble choosing words (1) (had this in the past).

Temperature is okay; averse heat of sun (2) now.

Voice and swallowing are okay.

Hair and scalp are better.

Desires sweets (3), breads and cereals (2), and ice cream (2).

Thirst is low (1). Wants colder drinks now.

Physical Examination: T4 = 3.8.

Assessment: Her energy is better, she is better on waking, her throat is better, and there is increasing initial sleeplessness, which is not quite similar to the previous condition. Anther change is an increased desire for sweets. My impression is that Magnesia muriatica has exerted a partial action, not being the exact simillimum at this time, and that a new remedy image is developing but is not yet apparent.

Plan: No remedy now.

Another Remedy is Needed

October 3, 1988

"I feel that I have different symptoms at different times."

Her scalp and skin are dry again (1).

On rainy days she wakens with a rough and swollen feeling in the throat and a deep, raspy voice (3); this improves later in the day. Constriction in the throat (1). Dysphagia in the morning with anything, solid or liquid (2).

Soreness of muscles lingers after any bump or straining (2).

Energy is fairly good. But it plummets during cold, wet weather (3).

Overall, not so chilly now. Cold hands and feet (2); worse from drafts (1). Little perspiration (3), even with exertion.

Concentration seems better; fades less easily. Better at choosing words.

Anxiety for loved ones (1).

Difficulty falling asleep due to mental alertness (2); no longer restless. Dreams of disasters (fire, losing people, broken relationships) (2). Sleeps on her abdomen or right side; she actually prefers the left, but suffers soreness of the left shoulder when lying on that side. Sleeps covered up.

Desires sweets (2), breads (2), ice cream (3), and milk (1).

Thirstless (2).

Gums are red and swollen.

Menses are only now recurring (she is weaning her baby). They come every five weeks.

No hand clumsiness.

Jaw is okay.

Analysis for the Next Prescription

Here is a clear change of remedy image. She is now clearly worse from cold and wet in general; she has a local aggravation of throat symptoms (hoarse in the morning and in wet weather); and she experiences soreness after straining her muscles.

I chose the following symptoms for repertorization:

1.	GENERALITIES:	Wet weather
2.	GENERALITIES:	Cold, aggravated, wet weather
3.	STOMACH:	Desires, ice cream
4.	STOMACH:	Desires, sweets

5. STOMACH: Desires, bread
6. STOMACH: Thirstless
7. SLEEP: Sleeplessness, thoughts, from
8. FEVER: Perspiration, absent
9. LARYNX: Voice, hoarseness, wet weather aggravates
10. LARYNX: Voice, hoarseness, morning
11. LARYNX: Voice, rough
12. LARYNX: Voice and Speech, aggravated, wet weather
13. LARYNX: Voice and Speech, aggravated, air, damp
14. THROAT: Pain, sore throat, damp weather
15. THROAT: Roughness, wet weather
16. EXTERNAL THROAT: Goiter
17. EXTERNAL THROAT: Goiter, constriction

Admittedly, this is a lot of symptoms to repertorize; nonetheless, let's see what comes up. It should be no surprise.

10/88 – totality

	Calc.	Ars.	Puls.	Lyc.	Phos.	Sulph.	Sil.	Carb-v.	Nat-m.	Am-c.	Bell.	Hep.
Total	25	21	21	20	19	19	18	15	15	14	14	14
Rubrics	10	9	9	10	10	9	10	8	9	8	8	8
Generalities; WET; weather												
Generalities; COLD; agg.; wet weather												
Stomach; DESIRES; ice cream												
Stomach; DESIRES; sweets												
Stomach; DESIRES; bread												
Stomach; THIRSTLESS												
Sleep; SLEEPLESSNESS; thoughts, from												
Fever; PERSPIRATION; absent												
Larynx; VOICE; hoarseness; wet;...												
Larynx; VOICE; hoarseness; morning												
Larynx; VOICE; rough												
Larynx; Voice and speech; AGG.; Wet;...												
Larynx; Voice and speech; AGG.; Air;...												
Throat; PAIN; Sorethroat; damp...												
Throat; ROUGHNESS; wet weather												
External Throat; GOITRE												
External Throat; GOITRE; constriction												

10/88 – totality; strange, rare, peculiar; small remedies; keynotes

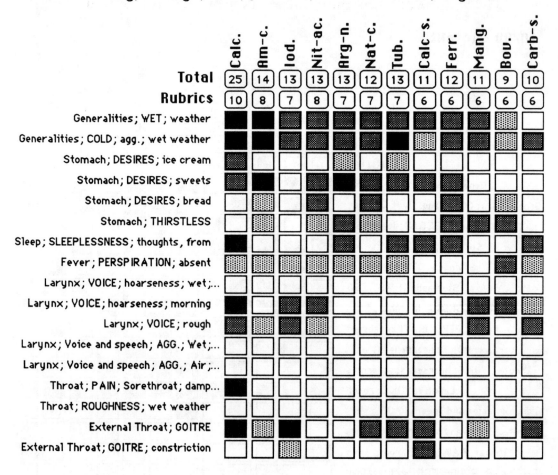

	Calc.	Am-c.	Iod.	Nit-ac.	Arg-n.	Nat-c.	Tub.	Calc-s.	Ferr.	Mang.	Bou.	Carb-s.
Total	25	14	13	13	13	12	13	11	12	11	9	10
Rubrics	10	8	7	8	7	7	7	6	6	6	6	6

Generalities; WET; weather
Generalities; COLD; agg.; wet weather
Stomach; DESIRES; ice cream
Stomach; DESIRES; sweets
Stomach; DESIRES; bread
Stomach; THIRSTLESS
Sleep; SLEEPLESSNESS; thoughts, from
Fever; PERSPIRATION; absent
Larynx; VOICE; hoarseness; wet;...
Larynx; VOICE; hoarseness; morning
Larynx; VOICE; rough
Larynx; Voice and speech; AGG.; Wet;...
Larynx; Voice and speech; AGG.; Air;...
Throat; PAIN; Sorethroat; damp...
Throat; ROUGHNESS; wet weather
External Throat; GOITRE
External Throat; GOITRE; constriction

So, Calcarea carbonica again comes up strongly, and this time the symptomatology much more clearly indicates it. Arsenicum album, Pulsatilla, Ammonium carbonicum, Sulphur, Silicea, and others bear little or no similarity to the case. Lycopodium has similarities but cannot compare to Calcarea. This patient sleeps on the right side, avoiding the left side because of the shoulder pain. Lycopodium is just the opposite: sleeps on the right side, and the shoulder pain is better lying on the painful side. The thirstlessness of the patient tends to exclude Phosphorus.

Plan: Calcarea carbonica 200c (Quinn).

Results of the Second Calcarea Carbonica Prescription

December 15, 1989

Feels less energetic (not underlined).

Frequent waking during the night (2); goes back to sleep easily; falls asleep easily now. No disaster dreams. Some trouble waking in the morning (1).

Flatulence after eating; also after drinking, even water (2). No bloating.

Is now okay during cold, wet weather. Cold feet (1).

Throat has been much better in the mornings; also has noted no difficulty with it during rainy weather.

No strained feeling in muscles. Side she lies on at night feels numb (3).

Energy is okay until early afternoon (2); better from a nap. Very weary by 4 p.m. (2); irritable and desires sweets (2) then. Is better by 9 p.m.

Scant perspiration (3).

Word choice is better; concentration is better.

No clumsiness of hands.

No taste for wine now. Desires sweets (3) and breads (2).

Low thirst.

Physical Examination:
- Her thyroid is still diffusely enlarged, mild.
- Weight = 147 lbs (a total weight loss of 14 pounds).
- Lab: T4 = 6.1!

Assessment: Despite her current complaint of lower energy (delivered with little emphasis), it is obvious that the remedy has had a salutary effect. Essentially, all symptoms are better, and the T4 has taken a big jump for the better. Of special interest is that when the Calcarea carbonica 10M (Quinn) was initially given, it did not act. It took Magnesia muriatica first, to remove a layer (improving thyroid function in the process) and to further clarify the Calcarea layer underneath. This experience should dispel the assertion of some homeopaths that the "constitutional remedy" is the only remedy that is ever required in a patient.

Plan: Wait

The Calcarea Carbonica is Repeated

March 13, 1989

She has noted again that rainy days make her mopey; she must force herself to be active (2).

Can concentrate better when reading, although she is sleepy when reading (3).

Energy is good in general; some slump in the early afternoon.

Is exercising.

Right arm goes to sleep at night (3), regardless of position. Prefers to sleep on left side (2). Sleep is generally good.

Cold feet at night (3); dry.

Normal perspiration.

Cold hands (1). Dry hands (2) for the past week on the sides of the fingers and the tips.

Normal temperature sensitivity.

Photophobia to the sunlight (3).

Early morning is her best time of day!

Desires farinaceous (2), sweets (1), cheese (2) and milk (1).

Thirsty for fruit juices.

Menses are more regular.

Physical Examination:
- Weight up to 152 lbs.
- Lab: T4 = 5.5.

Assessment: While she is still better than before taking the Calcarea carbonica, there are signs of slipping: weight is up, energy is down (during interim, had noted more energy in general), T4 is down, and the sensitivity to rainy weather has returned. Some symptoms have shifted: craving for sweets is less, perspiration is more normal, thirst is up, and sleeps on the left side (was able to return to this preferred position when her shoulder was no longer too sore). But there is no major shift in the symptom pattern. It is appropriate therefore to represcribe the remedy, although one couldn't be faulted for opting to wait.

Plan: Calcarea carbonica 200c (Quinn)

Steady Improvement: Lab Values Begin to Normalize

May 2, 1989

Felt great until her daughter was bitten by a dog; since then, she has felt anxious, experiencing recurring images of her daughter's bitten face; also anxious at night; self-reproach.

Energy is good; a little slow to start on rainy days.

Arm is not numb now.

No cold feet.

Hands are less dry.

Desires farinaceous (3).

Thirsty (2).

Assessment: The patient is better.

Plan: Wait.

June 1989

Lab: T4 = 6.2.

September 19, 1989

Generally feels quite well.

On one rainy day, she had low energy.

Phlegm in throat for one week.

Desires sweets and farinaceous.

Thirsty.

Appetite is high in the morning.

Sleep is quite good.

Eyes are slightly sensitive to light.

Skin texture is normal.

Lab:
- T4 = 10.7.
- TSH = 10.7 (down from 50).

Assessment: Her thyroid is functioning at upper levels of normal; the TSH will normalize. The continued sensitivity to wet weather and persistent food cravings suggest that Calcarea carbonica will continue to be her remedy if she relapses. (There have been hints that Lycopodium may at some time surface as well.)

Now, she remains essentially well.

Here is this patient's clinical course depicted graphically (plotting the T4 values on the y axis and the sequence of remedies on the x axis):

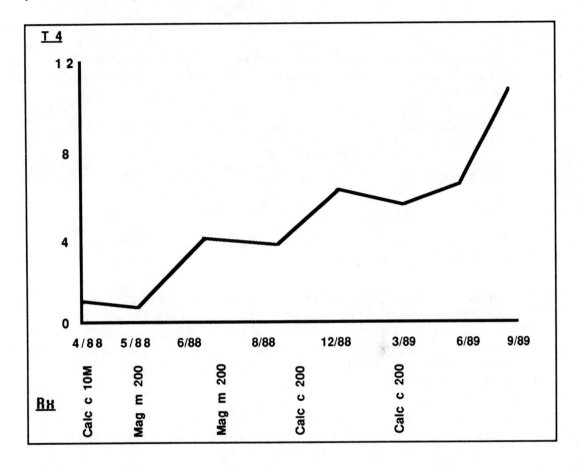

Guess: Before I make some general comments on the treatment of hypothyroidism, do you have any questions?

Audience: Had there been any thyroid supplementation in this case?

Guess: No. Fortunately she was treated early.

Audience: Often postpartum women will have a certain degree of hypothyroidism and then will feel better after they wean. I was wondering how you felt her weaning fit into this change.

Guess: It may have given her a final boost, but the graph clearly demonstrates a correlation between improvement in the T4 values and the remedies given. I checked the medical literature, and I couldn't find a clear association between a transient profound hypothyroidism and the postnatal period. There is an entity called subclinical thyroiditis, in which a transient hypothyroidism follows a period of preliminary hyperthyroidism. I did question this patient about her pregnancy but couldn't elicit any hint of a symptom of hyperthyroidism.

Murray Feldman: I was wondering if you saw any etiological factors other than the postpartum?

Guess: No.

Murray Feldman: What about the domestic situation? Was there anything there?

Guess: No. The home life was normal.

Teresa Salvadore: Whitmont, in his book Psyche and Substance, *has a nice comparative study between Magnesia muriatica and Calcarea carbonica. He says that both remedies are strongly focused on the theme of responsibility and can become quite anxious about it. But Calcarea carbonica goes easily into a state of exhaustion, while Magnesia muriatica goes more easily into a state of restlessness. This case makes me wonder if the two remedies could be complementary.*

Guess: Well, that may be new information we can develop, and this case might give further credence to Whitmont's ideas.

Vithoulkas, in his materia medica on Magnesia muriatica, talks about the confusion between Magnesia muriatica and Rhus toxicodendron, because of that nocturnal restlessness. But Magnesia muriatica can be aggravated by milk, where we know that Rhus toxicodendron has a strong craving for it. He suggests that the milk be used as a possible differential point, although it wouldn't have helped in this case.

Comments on Treating Hypothyroid
Patients Who Are on Thyroid Supplementation

In the case I just described, the patient was not taking any conventional thyroid supplementation. However, because many patients are on thyroid supplementation when they come to see us, a few comments on this situation may be of interest.

Patients can respond to homeopathic remedies while on thyroid supplementation (such as Synthroid). For example, a congenital hypothyroid case will respond to each homeopathic dose with a decrease in TSH and an improvement in symptoms, with each dose generating a progressively longer effect. Thus, it is possible not only to produce positive symptomatic changes but also to actually have a beneficial effect on the thyroid condition itself.

Patients on thyroid supplements definitely will respond to remedies given for other, nonthyroid conditions. One such patient, who came in for arthritis, allergies, and other problems, was diagnosed years ago as having hypothyroidism and has been on Synthroid ever since.

While these overlaid conditions do respond, my impression is that the extent of clinical improvement in these patients is less than optimal. I feel that, at some point in the course of treatment, the need to address the hypothyroid state with homeopathic remedies arises; however, if the patient continues on thyroid supplementation, the clinical indications for deeper treatment never surface, leaving the practitioner capable of providing only more superficial, palliative treatment. If the patient can be convinced to abandon his Synthroid, greater gains are possible, but not always assured (especially after decades of thyroid suppression).

Other practitioners I polled felt that patients on thyroid supplementation relapse earlier, in general being more clinically labile; that they are in general more difficult to treat; and that the longer they have been on thyroid supplementation, the harder they are to treat and the more difficult it is to wean them off the supplements.

Different practitioners have different methods for managing these cases. One prefers to discontinue the thyroid supplementation, prescribe a placebo, re-evaluate the case in six weeks, and then prescribe the indicated homeopathic remedy. Another physician leaves his patients on the thyroid and immediately initiates homeopathic treatment, reducing the thyroid supplementation once the patients show a response. The success of this method obviously is dependent upon the accuracy of the symptom image available at the initial interview. If no clear image is apparent, it is preferable to discontinue the thyroid supplement for four to six weeks, then re-evaluate the case.

It is generally agreed that a thyroid supplement can be discontinued for about one month before the symptoms of hypothyroidism definitely begin to reassert themselves; during that month there is little danger to the patient. Obviously the extent to which the patient's thyroid function is compromised will determine how wise it is to extend the period of abstinence from supplementation while awaiting a curative response to homeopathic treatment.

As you know, many patients have been incorrectly placed on thyroid supplements in the past and, after an initial adjustment period subsequent to its withdrawal, will do quite well without. The principal danger of withdrawal from thyroid supplementation is, of course, the precipitation of myxedema coma (usually occurring after some significant stress, such as an acute febrile condition). Additionally, in children, withdrawal from thyroid supplements may compromise physical growth, physical maturation, and mental development.

Guess: Do other people have observations on treating patients on thyroid supplementation, or on hypothyroid patients in general?

Michael Carlston: I've treated quite a few cases. Many of these have been what I call "factitious" hypothyroidism, because the patients were not truly hypothyroid but were put on thyroid supplementation as a stimulant to their general energy. In these and in the true cases of hypothyroidism I have never seen any problem with treating people who are on thyroid supplementation. Most of them have been able to stop the thyroid medication or certainly reduce it quite a bit.

Guess: I would like to emphasize one point regarding children with hypothyroidism. A number of these cases may stem from a congenital absence of a thyroid gland. I had a pediatric case that was not responding, but the parents did not want the child on thyroid medication. I realized at some point that he had never had a scan. I ordered one, and, in fact, the child had no thyroid. So, it's important to have a proper medical evaluation, especially in pediatric age groups. They certainly won't respond if they don't have a gland.

Jonathan Shore: One warning. Many years ago I had a patient who was hypothyroid and was on thyroid medication. I gave her Lachesis, which acted *very nicely. She didn't return for follow-up because of financial constraints. About two or three months later she ended up in the emergency room in hyperthyroid crisis because I had neglected to tell her to stop her thyroid medication as her health improved.*

Guess: A word to the wise.

Teresa Salvadore: I had a similar experience with Lachesis. The patient had been on thyroid medication for many years, and it was necessary to stop the medication after the remedy was given. She was having heart palpitations from the excess thyroid. The other case I wanted to bring up was a case of Hashimoto's thyroiditis that had been medicated for a year. The patient went into Hashimoto's one week after the death of her father. This turned out to be a Causticum case, and, after I gave her the Causticum, she immediately developed an intense sore throat and swollen glands that would go right to left, left to right, right to left, and so on. We waited one week, as long as she could handle it. I finally gave her Lac caninum, and her energy immediately increased more than it had ever been on the thyroid medication. We eventually weaned her off the thyroid medication, and she is doing fine. One last note. When her alternating sore throats did go away she got a rash in the shape of a butterfly on the outside of her throat, over the thyroid area. I thought this was a nice healing reaction.

Guess: A beautiful case.

Sheryl R. Kipnis, ND, DHANP

TWO CASES
OF PRIMARY
HYPERTHYROIDISM

Sheryl Kipnis, ND, DHANP, is a graduate of the National College of Naturopathic Medicine. She is board-certified in homeopathy by the Homeopathic Academy of Naturopathic Physicians (HANP) and is a past member of the HANP Board of Directors. Sheryl has been teaching in the IFH Professional Course since 1985. She is a co-founder of the Ravenna Homeopathic Clinic, Seattle, Washington, where she maintains a private practice specializing in homeopathy.

Introduction

Homeopathy is really remarkable! The standard allopathic treatment for primary hyperthyroidism includes use of drugs (mostly Propylthiouracil), radioactive iodine, or surgery — all aimed at suppressing the activity of the thyroid gland. These treatments carry their own risks and possible side effects, and sometimes leave the patient in a chronically hypothyroid state. Radioiodine therapy and surgery are said to be among the most common causes for chronic hypothyroidism. But how incredible to be able to give a few granules of nontoxic medication to patients, and then have their own bodies bring things back into balance; to resolve the hyperthyroid state, without the subsequent risk of developing hypothyroidism; and to bring the person as a whole to a greater level of health!

I have with me today two cases from my practice, actually the only two cases of primary hyperthyroidism that I have seen in my eight years of practice. I think these cases are interesting for a couple of reasons. The first, perhaps, is that these cases are well documented in terms of blood tests that reflect both the original diagnosis and the resolution of the disease. Many of us successfully treat a lot of illnesses that cannot be diagnosed or documented, so there are no objective data to show that the remedies prescribed actually did something. Homeopaths are often accused of having only anecdotes to tell; it is suggested that patients want to get better and so they report that they are better, with no objective proof of their healing.

The other reason these cases are of interest to me is *because* of the lab work. It is interesting to look at how the blood tests may or may not reflect the degree of healing that is taking place. I will be interested to know if others here have made similar observations in their own practices.

Case Number 1

Female
Age 32
Bookkeeper

Description of the Patient

The first case is that of a 32-year-old woman. She came in because she was getting frequent colds in the last year or more, and she wondered if she might be hyperthyroid. There was a strong family history of hyperthyroidism on the mother's side of the family: The patient's mother, grandmother, and aunt were hyperthyroid. She had noticed a change in her health sometime in the last year, although she wasn't really sure when the symptoms first began.

The patient is fair-skinned, with red hair. She is rather plain looking, and has a generally unkempt appearance. Most of the time, she wears army green work pants, flannel or tee shirts, and some sort of work boot. There is a musty odor about her that is always present, like the smell of clothing that has been stored in a trunk in the attic for 20 years. The odor remains in the office long after she is gone. Her voice is very small and child-like, and her answers are vague. She tends to not be very observant of herself, telling me that she just doesn't pay that much attention to the details. If she has pain, she takes a pill and then she can forget about the pain.

She is five feet, four inches tall and weighs 140 pounds.

Family History:
- Mother: hyperthyroid, hypertension, cancer.
- Brother: skin cancer.
- Maternal Aunt: hyperthyroid.
- Maternal grandmother: hyperthyroid.

Patient History: 1984 laparoscopy for infertility, diagnosed as endometriosis. Has a two-year-old adopted son.

January 5, 1989

The patient came to see me for the initial visit, and reported the following:

Her nose is always stuffed; her throat is frequently sore (2). Lately, her nose dries up, and she gets a headache (2) around the sinus area. In winter, one cold follows on the heels of the previous one.

She used to get migraines. Now she gets them only once or twice a year, lasting about three days each time. Rarely severe. Pain starts on the right side, moves to the whole head, and finishes on the left side. The headache is sometimes worse when eating (1), sometimes triggered by cold and bright light (1). Has a similar kind of pain when the sun is shining through the trees as she is driving (1).

(*Very* restless legs.)

She has been losing weight lately. Had gained weight in the past year, from 130 to over 140 pounds. Now is down to mid 130s. Hasn't been especially hungry in the mornings and is eating less.

Feet are more restless than previously (2). Was very tense in high school, then calmed down a lot.

Itchy (2) around her neck lately, without eruption. Acne on chest in last several years.

Warm (2) normally, and notices no significant change in body temperature lately.

On going to bed at night, has noticed that her pulse is high. Feels like her heart is pounding (2), although it doesn't keep her awake. Pulse is normally 70 to 80 beats per minute. Hasn't taken her pulse when she feels it is racing.

Sleep is generally good and sound, although she is tired on waking because she stays up too late. Often wants to stay in bed, "a mid-day person." Feels best 8 a.m. to 10 p.m. Sleeps on left side (1). Salivates only with naps. Feet are not outside the covers. No grinding of teeth; no night sweats; no nightmares.

Has one adopted child. Looking to adopt another. She has endometriosis, which was treated in 1984 with electrocautery. Has been trying to conceive for five years, without success. No clear explanation for her infertility. Whenever she wants to do something, she makes it happen (2). It is difficult for her to realize she can't control everything (2).

Fears: "Boogie people in my room at night" — all her life (2). Had to change sides of the bed with her husband so that she would not have to sleep on the outside edge, because of her fear. Fears falling when on a high place (2).

Worries a lot (2). If her husband is late, she imagines him dead on the highway. Worries about her health and her child. "I can take care of everything while worrying."

Wants to control everything around her, to have control in her life. For example, nags her husband (2), telling him to do things when *she* thinks they should be done. Confronts very few people; mostly her husband. May feel angry at housemate, but nags at husband instead. Nags herself (2); tells herself she is a bad person for getting angry and nagging others.

She was the youngest in a family of four. "A painfully normal family." Father yelled a lot, but not abusive.

Feels torn between the "should" to have a career and the desire to have a family. When wanting a career, feels she is not a good mother (tears) because she yells at her son a lot, which she learned from her father.

Worries about her relationship with her husband. He doesn't communicate well (2). Feels like a failure (2) on both sides, because she has no real career and can't stay at home all the time.

Low interest in sex (2) since first trying to get pregnant, and then again after adopting their son. Is too tired. At 18, she was "obsessed" with sex. Had sex every day with her first lover. Masturbated every night when around ten years old. Experimented sexually with women in high school. Could have gone either way sexually.

Menses are regular. Often severe cramps. Unable to describe the symptoms because she takes Motrin every month as soon as the pain begins. Sometimes has migraines with the period.

Pain in the urethra once a week, with urging to urinate, or sometimes after urination. Began about six months ago. Feels a sensation that travels upwards, and then is gone.

Appetite and digestion are good. Lots of foul gas (2), which comes and goes and is worse before menses.

Desires popcorn (2), sweets (3), fish (1), and rich cheesy foods.
Likes crisp fat (1), "I like fatty meat!"

Averse to beets (2), green peppers (2), and fried eggs (2).

Thirsty (2). Lips are dry on waking. Keeps water by the bed. Ice is okay; dislikes extremely hot drinks.

Generally worse around 2 or 3 p.m.

Physical Examination: Her thyroid is moderately enlarged, smooth, and boggy. No nodules palpated.

Lab:
- T4 RIA = 15.5 (normal = 4.5-12.5).
- T3U = 38.4 (normal = 22.0-35.0).
- T3 RIA = 300 (normal = 80-200).
- FTI = 5.95 (normal = 1.3-3.9).
- SGOT = 52 (normal = 0-40).
- SGPT = 95 (normal = 0-45).
- Hematocrit = 36.8 (normal = 37.0-47.0).
- HDL Cholesterol = 52 (normal > 55).
- Cholesterol = 159 (normal = 130-200).
- All other lab work was within normal limits.

Analysis of Case Number 1

I'm afraid the analysis of this case is not terribly profound. (Or, maybe it is profound in its simplicity.) It was a case that frustrated me. First of all, I was frustrated in the taking of the case. The lack of specific information left me feeling that I might just as well close my eyes and randomly select a remedy from my pharmacy! I knew that I would have to study the case because I didn't have a clue about what to give this woman while I was with her. I also knew that, once I sat down to study the case, the lack of information was still going to frustrate me. What is there to study?

Nonetheless, study I did. I turned on the computer and hoped that MacRepertory would shed some light. (All computer analyses were generated using MacRepertory 3.4, from Kent Homeopathic Associates.) I entered symptoms into each of the three clipboards. In the first clipboard, I put the hyperthyroid symptoms, which were very few and general: goiter, swelling of the thyroid, palpitations at night in bed, and restlessness of the lower limbs. These were the only symptoms she had observed since the condition began, without any other modalities or concomitant symptoms. I put her other complaints into the second clipboard, and her general symptoms into the third clipboard.

The complete list of symptoms is as follows:

1.	EXTERNAL THROAT:	Goiter
2.	EXTERNAL THROAT:	Thyroid gland
3.	EXTREMITIES:	Restlessness, lower limbs
4.	CHEST:	Palpitation heart, night, bed, in
5.	GENERALITIES:	Cold, tendency to take
6.	NOSE:	Catarrh, dry, chronic
7.	HEAD PAIN:	Localization, sides, right, then left
8.	HEAD PAIN:	General, eating, after
9.	HEAD PAIN:	General, cold, becoming, from
10.	HEAD PAIN:	General, light, from, light in general
11.	FEMALE GENITALIA:	Sterility
12.	FEMALE GENITALIA:	Menses, painful, dysmenorrhoea
13.	URETHRA:	Pain, urging to urinate, on
14.	URETHRA:	Pain, urination, after
15.	SLEEP:	Position, side, on, left
16.	GENERALITIES:	Warm, aggravated
17.	MIND:	Fear, robbers, of
18.	MIND:	Fear, falling, of
19.	FEMALE GENITALIA:	Desire, diminished
20.	STOMACH:	Desires, sweets
21.	STOMACH:	Desires, fish
22.	STOMACH:	Desires, fat
23.	GENERALITIES:	Afternoon, 2 p.m.
24.	GENERALITIES:	Afternoon, 3 p.m.

In looking only at the hyperthyroid symptoms, the obvious remedy, Iodium, is suggested. It's probably one of the first remedies a homeopath thinks of when hyperthyroid is mentioned: restlessness, racing heart, big appetite, weight loss, swelling and induration of glands, and easily overheated. So, I looked at it and tried to make it fit the case. But, try as I might, I just couldn't convince myself. The symptoms of her disease were very general and common, and not really strong enough for Iodium. In addition, there wasn't anything in the case that clearly made it Iodium. She didn't describe having a ravenous appetite and losing weight in spite of eating large amounts. She also didn't describe the forgetfulness of Iodium or the impulse to do violence.

Polycrest remedies such as Sulphur and Causticum were suggested, but I couldn't make enough of a case for either of these remedies.

Looking for a peculiar or outstanding symptom in a case is often a good strategy. The pain in her urethra is about as close to peculiar as I could find. The remedies in the rubric URETHRA, pain, on urging to urinate include Agaricus, Cocculus, Conium, and Hypericum. None of these remedies fit the patient or the pathology very well.

If I step back from the case, I see a woman who is very restless, very anxious, and very fearful. She has an intense fear of someone breaking into the house, so strong that she made her husband change sides of the bed with her! In addition to this, she likes fat. These symptoms suggest Arsenicum album, but she is warm. In addition, Arsenicum album is not a remedy especially known for its usefulness in treating a patient with hyperthyroidism. Iodium is, however. Using MacRepertory to analyze these symptoms, one can see that both Arsenicum album and Iodium are strongly suggested.

So, I combined these two elements and looked at Arsenicum iodatum. I would love to lead you to some obscure rubric in the repertory, unique to the case, where Arsenicum iodatum is strongly represented, but I just couldn't find it. Actually, there is good reason for this. Arsenicum iodatum is in the repertory only 915 times, contrasted with Arsenicum album, which appears 6,194 times, and Iodium, which appears 2,219 times!

As I read about Arsenicum iodatum, I discovered that one of the more significant problems associated with this remedy is the tendency to get colds often, resulting in much nasal stuffiness and discharge. Kent describes a lot of nasal catarrh, nasal obstruction, dryness in the nose, and pain in the head from catarrh of the nasal

Repertorization of the January 1989 case:

Totality	Small Remedies	Strange, Rare &	Symptom Strength	Keynotes	Number of Rubrics
58 Iod.	31 Merc-i-r.	8 Puls.	58 Iod.	27 Ars.	75 Bell.
50 Ars.	30 Sanic.	7 Sulph.	50 Ars.	27 Puls.	75 Iod.
50 Puls.	28 Ail.	6 Iod.	50 Puls.	25 Sulph.	75 Mag-c.
49 Nat-m.	23 Aur-i.	5 Rhus-t.	49 Nat-m.	18 Iod.	75 Nat-c.
49 Sil.	23 Calc-i.	4 Ars.	49 Sil.	15 Calc.	75 Nat-m.
41 Lyc.	22 Aml-n.	4 Ox-ac.	41 Lyc.	15 Spong.	75 Sil.
41 Rhus-t.	22 Aur-s.	4 Ph-ac.	41 Rhus-t.	4 Lyc.	50 Ail.
41 Tarent.	22 Jal.	4 Spig.	41 Tarent.	4 Nat-m.	50 Alum.
41 Zinc.	22 Lap-a.	3 Ferr.	41 Zinc.	4 Rhus-t.	50 Ars.
33 Caust.	22 Sol-t-ae.	3 Lach.	33 Caust.	4 Sil.	50 Aur.
33 Ferr.	22 Zinc-p.	3 Nat-m.	33 Ferr.	4 Tarent.	50 Caust.
33 Lach.	20 Calc-f.	3 Phos.	33 Lach.	4 Zinc.	50 Con.
33 Nat-c.	19 Iod.	3 Sil.	33 Nat-c.	3 Caust.	50 Ferr.
33 Phos.	19 Urt-u.	3 Zinc.	33 Phos.	3 Ferr.	50 Graph.
33 Stram.	18 Bad.	2 Arg-n.	33 Stram.	3 Lach.	50 Kali-c.
33 Sulph.	18 Cimx.	2 Aur.	33 Sulph.	3 Phos.	50 Lach.
25 Calc.	18 Lycps.	2 Cact.	25 Calc.	3 Stram.	50 Lyc.
25 Chin.	18 Ox-ac.	2 Con.	25 Chin.	2 Ail.	50 Merc.
25 Kali-br.	17 Kali-br.	2 Ign.	25 Kali-br.	2 Alum.	50 Merc-i-r.
25 Nux-v.	16 Carl.	2 Lyc.	25 Nux-v.	2 Aur.	50 Ox-ac.
25 Spong.	16 Tarent.	2 Merc.	25 Spong.	2 Chin.	50 Phos.
24 Ail.	15 Arum-t.	2 Nat-c.	24 Ail.	2 Con.	50 Plat.

passages. Arsenicum iodatum has many iodine characteristics: swelling and induration of various glands, a small and rapid pulse, and aggravation from heat. It is a remedy known for having a lot of anxiety and restlessness, relating to both the iodine and the arsenic elements.

Last year, when I spoke at this conference, I presented a case of Natrum arsenicosum, and I described the process of prescribing a remedy that is a salt or "combination" of two other remedies. I talked about how the patient might have elements of one remedy and elements of another, not clearly being one or the other. And I stated that, in order to give the "combination" remedy with confidence, it was important to have at least one keynote that belonged to the salt itself. In this case, I wasn't able to find such a keynote. I gave the remedy anyway, but not with overwhelming confidence.

When taking a case, I sometimes find myself getting frustrated with a patient if there isn't a lot of information forthcoming. I feel that I don't have much to prescribe on. One thing I learned from this case was that, although there wasn't much information, there was enough. In its infinite wisdom, the body somehow manages to bring out what is truly important, and it falls to me to accept this and not force the issue. She was a woman whose symptoms included hyperthyroidism, fear and anxiety, and getting colds frequently: Iodium plus Arsenicum album leading to Arsenicum iodatum!

Results of Arsenicum Iodatum Prescription in Case Number 1

I will be brief on the follow-up, because I would like to get to the second case. I gave her one dose of Arsenicum iodatum 200c. I saw her four weeks later, and her first statement was "I feel great...wonderful...lots better!" She had lots of energy and was very active. Her resting pulse had remained up around 100 beats per minute until one week before the follow-up visit and then dropped to around 80, where it had remained. Her weight had continued to drop, to 125 pounds, and then increased again to 133, where it had stabilized.

Her restlessness was much less, and, because of this, she was able to be more productive. She sat and sewed last night for the first time in a long time. Her menses was very mild. She was anxious about not taking Motrin during her period but found that she didn't need it. She had a cold just before taking the remedy. Her nose had been stuffy for the last couple of weeks, but the cold was beginning to resolve.

She had no palpitations at night. She couldn't recall sitting around worrying lately, and was nagging her husband less. Her sexual interest had increased. She was feeling less conflicted about working versus staying home. She hadn't noticed fear at night for a while.

On examination, I found that her pulse was 92, blood pressure was 120/58, heart sounds were normal, and the thyroid gland was unchanged.

She continued to improve over the next year. Her subjective hyperthyroid symptoms were completely gone shortly after the first follow-up visit. She continued having frequent colds for a while, but they gradually tapered off. She never had another dose of the remedy.

In June 1989, I repeated the blood tests. This was five months after the remedy had been given. Her T4 had decreased from 15.5 to 13.1. Her T3 had decreased from 300 to 230. Both were still above normal. I found this interesting in light of the fact that her subjective hyperthyroid symptoms had been absent for many months. Her hematocrit and liver enzymes had returned to normal. Her cholesterol had increased from 152 to 206, but, with that, her HDL had increased. So, she actually had a lower risk of heart disease (according to statistics, anyway) than previously.

In January 1990, I once again repeated the blood tests and found her T4 was 8.6 and her T3 was 119, both well within the limits of normal. Because I was doing blood tests only every six months, it was difficult to know when the hormones actually returned to normal. But I find it interesting that it apparently took place quite a few months after the overt symptoms of the disease resolved.

Case Number 2

Female
Age 29
Oyster Farmer

The second case is that of a 29-year-old woman who worked as an oyster farmer. She was much more overtly hyperthyroid than the woman in the first case, and the blood tests reflected this. She was fair-skinned and blonde, very red in the face, and chubby. She was quite restless and spoke quickly and excitedly.

Family History:
- Father: died of a heart attack at age 63.
- Mother: nervous breakdown.
- Paternal grandmother: goiter.

Patient History: Mononucleosis when 21 years old. Allergic to aspirin.

May 12, 1986

The patient came to see me for hyperthyroid problems, and reported the following:

Her symptoms began a couple of months ago: heart beating fast, swelling of tibias, and feeling weak and shaky. Was diagnosed hyperthyroid: "thyroxine was twice the normal level"; EKG was normal. Symptoms began after a two-day fast with lemon, honey, and cayenne.

Legs are normal in the morning on waking. By mid-morning they start swelling, with pitting edema. Feet also used to swell in the beginning, but no longer.

Hot all the time (3). Temperature before illness was average or chilly. Never chilly now! Desires open air (3) since the illness began. Likes to sprawl out because it is cooler.

Heart is always fast (2), and has shaking in extremities (2). Heart and throat sometimes feel hollow (2), several times a day, like a column from mid-chest to throat (2).

Nervousness is more extreme than would normally be in new situations.

Sighs often (2). (Sighs frequently throughout the interview.)

Has bitten her nails all her life.

Difficult to get up in the morning (2). Feels drowsy (2). Feels stiff (2) all over on waking. Soles of feet are sore (2); floor feels too hard on bare feet (2). Legs also become stiff after long period of sitting (2).

Sleep is poor; restless (2); tosses and turns (2) in sleep. Sometimes wakes with heart racing; sleeps through the night or wakes once. Prefers sleeping on side (2) or abdomen (2). Rarely salivates; perspires (2); feet are covered.

Back itches (2) (many small moles and birthmarks; some pimples). Worse later in the day; better from scratching and rubbing (2).

Short of breath on slight exertion (2), as if she's severely obese. Heavy work causes a cramp (2) in her right hypochondrium (2), occasionally in the left: comes on quickly, has to stop work, lasts five minutes; cramp in one spot only; sometimes doubles over from the cramp; subsides at rest, and returns if she resumes work.

Fatigue (2); becomes upset and cries because can't work hard. Then husband gets upset with her for not working and yells at her. Not as much of a problem now that she and husband both know why she is so tired and weak. Feels frustrated and angry. Sometimes gets really angry (2) with husband. He incited a mean dog around her and she hit him (tears). Husband gets wild ideas and talks excitedly about his ideas. She feels no control over what will happen in their life and gets upset. An ongoing problem for past six years, since they have been together. Husband is extremely idealistic and tries to impose this on her.

Lives a very simple life on a houseboat. Only way to protest government is to not pay taxes, and only way to do this is to not earn much money. No desire for children: "too much commitment, too selfish."

Grew up with stepmother and father from age seven, after mother's breakdown. Stepmother was very controlling (2), especially over food eaten. So, whenever her stepmother went out, she would eat (3), vomit (2), and eat more (3). Still binge eats when husband goes out: "I can do anything I want."

Able to assert herself with husband but constantly has to struggle against him. Can't just relax and be herself. Not especially unhappy with her life.

Desires cereal and milk (2) (has desired these all her life; would hoard her favorites), chips (2), butter on foods (2), spicy (2), lemon (1), milk (1), French fries/ketchup (2), crunchy (2), and eggs.

Averse to clams/mussels (2), fat (2), and strong cheese (2).

Thirsty (3) for cold since illness began.

Digestion is good. Bowel movements three times per day since the fast; constipation all her life before the fast.

All her life felt she wasn't getting what she wanted, and not enough (2).

In college was binge eating and spending money out of control, although it was the happiest time in her life.

Sometimes becomes very fearful (2) that her mother will "flip out" and hurt her (2). Becomes angry (2) when scared: yells (2) and cries (1). Does things because she thinks they will be fun, such as going out on a boat in rough water, and then gets scared.

Feels unattractive; doesn't believe husband's compliments. Had an affair last year; ended last August; ending felt like a death (2). Her lover was married, and her husband insisted on telling the lover's wife. She and her husband have an open relationship. Still in love with this other man, although she never wanted to leave her husband. During the affair she got trichomoniasis. It was treated with antibiotics, and then she got a yeast infection. Still has occasional burning at the vaginal introitus.

Likes sex, but lacks excitement. Desire is average. Difficult to climax.

Menses are regular. Cramps the first day, sometimes very bad and causing diarrhea. Cramps are aggravated by coffee (2), eating (1), sitting; they are better when she is lying down.

Profuse perspiration (2), especially on face. Face flushes red (2) easily, especially with exertion. Feet sweat a lot, without strong odor.

She occasionally smokes cigarettes; craves them.

Physical Examination:
- Blood Pressure: 110/68.
- Pulse: 108.
- Heart: regular rate and rhythm; no extra sounds or murmurs.
- Thyroid: slightly enlarged, not tender, no nodules palpable.

Lab:
- T4 = 21.5 (normal = 4.5-12.5).
- T3U = 42.0 (normal = 23-34).
- Free T4 (calculated) = 9.12 (normal = 1.0-4.3).

- Cholesterol = 120 (normal = 125-202).
- Total Protein = 6.0 (normal = 6.4-8.0).
- Albumin = 3.6 (normal = 3.7-4.8).
- White Blood Count = 3.2 (normal = 3.9-11.4).
- Hemoglobin = 11.4 (normal 11.8-15.6).
- Hematocrit = 34.2 (normal = 35.0-46.0).

Analysis of Case Number 2

Analyzing this case was just the opposite situation from Case Number 1. Where the last case seemed to have a paucity of information, this case is almost overwhelming! So, once again, I turned to MacRepertory, looking at least for clues and a place to start. When I looked at the case as a whole, Sulphur (of course!) and Pulsatilla were equally and highly represented.

First Prescription and Follow-Up on Case Number 2

I chose to give her Pulsatilla, one dose of 200c. I made this decision for two reasons. First, it seemed to fit the specific symptoms of the case. Second, it seemed to fit the way she described herself in her life: a person easily influenced by those around her, unable to assert her own needs and desires. She was too thirsty for a Pulsatilla, but I didn't let that stop me.

June 1986

At the first follow-up visit about six weeks later, she reported some improvement. She noted that, for about three weeks after the remedy, she needed much more sleep, some days sleeping almost all day. This need had decreased in the last week or so. I am thrilled when a patient comes in with a story like this. I like nothing better than when patients call me after receiving a remedy and tell me how tired they are and how they are needing or wanting to sleep all the time. The body repairs itself during sleep. If someone has an overwhelming desire to sleep after being given a remedy, it is an indication to me that the remedy is having deep action and that healing is taking place. Her sleep was generally better. She was no longer restless, was not waking with a pounding heart, and felt rested on waking.

Repertorization of the May 1986 case:

	Sulph.	Puls.	Merc.	Phos.	Lyc.	Nat-m.	Ars.	Sil.	Calc.
Total	37	36	31	30	29	28	27	27	26
Rubrics	18	17	15	15	12	14	12	12	13
Generalities; AIR; open; desire for	3	3		1	3	2	2		
Generalities; WARM; agg.	2	3	2	2	2	2			
Respiration; DIFFICULT; exertion, after	2	2	2	2	3	3	3	2	3
Chest; EMPTINESS, sensation of	1								
Chest; PALPITATION heart	3	3	3	3	3	3	3	2	3
Extremities; SWELLING; Leg	1	2	2		3		3	3	2
Extremities; STIFFNESS; morning				2					
Extremity Pain; SORE; Foot; sole	1	2	1	1	1			2	1
Back; ITCHING	3	2	2	1	2	1		2	1
Mind; SIGHING	1	1				1			
Abdomen; PAIN; cramping	3	3	2	1	3	2	2	3	3
Face; DISCOLORATION; red	2	2	2	3	2	2	2	2	1
Sleep; UNREFRESHING	2	2		3	2	2	2	2	1
Stomach; DESIRES; butter		1	1						
Stomach; DESIRES; highly seasoned food	3	1		3					
Stomach; DESIRES; lemons			2			1	1		
Stomach; DESIRES; milk	1		2	2		2	2	2	2
Stomach; DESIRES; eggs		2						1	2
Stomach; AVERSION to; fats and rich food	2	3	2	1		2	2		1
Stomach; AVERSION to; cheese; strong...	2		2						
Stomach; THIRST; extreme	3	1	3	3	2	3	3	3	3
Face; PERSPIRATION	2	3	3	2	3	2	2	3	3

She was less hot overall. She still felt weak and shaky, but less so. She still felt a rapid heartbeat, but her heart was pounding less. Her resting pulse still averaged 110. She described an achy sensation in her external throat the last few days, like a cramp or knot, a swollen sensation. She described it as "almost like a sore throat, but not inside; it is a slight constriction, like a lump." She no longer noticed swelling in her feet. She was still short of breath on exertion, but not as much.

It was my clinical impression that she was improving, so I waited. Lab work was repeated in August: her T4 was unchanged, her T3U was at the upper limit of normal, her FTI had decreased some but was still elevated, and her T3 (which had not been tested previously) was 808! In addition to this, her liver enzymes and her glucose were elevated. Both of these had been normal previously. Her iron level was significantly elevated as well. I was greatly concerned about her T3 level. I consulted with a couple of internists who said they had never seen a T3 that high! Unfortunately, there was no way to know if it had been that high since the onset of her illness, or if it was increasing. However, because she had been in this hyperthyroid state for many months and her symptoms were gradually improving, the concern that she would go into thyroid storm was not very great. So, I was advised to watch her closely.

September 30, 1986

The patient was tearful.

Gets upset really easily (2). Easily frustrated and nervous, then becomes shaky (2) and tearful (2).

Her husband had an affair in July. She was much more upset than she thought she would be, then she was down on herself for being so upset (2). Really angry (3) with the woman. Yelled at her a couple of times (2). Doesn't want to see her ever (3)! Jealous (3). Believes if she felt better about herself, it wouldn't be so hard. Her husband is still friends with the woman, and the patient can't tolerate having her around. Feels jealous (2) and repulsed (2) by her. Dreams of being violent to her (2), cutting her with a knife. Feels persecuted by her (2).

In August, she spent all day walking in the hot sun at an international exposition, and felt her symptoms returning. Felt shaky (2), weak (2), and hot (2). Had to lie down in the first aid tent. Blood pressure was 140/90. Pulse varies generally from 90 to 110 or 120.

Desires open air (3). Can't sleep with windows closed (3), becomes hot and restless.

Tired (2). Some days worse than others. Even tired on waking in the morning, although sleep feels wonderful!

Aching stiffness (2) and sore soles (2) on rising from lying or sitting and in the morning on first stepping out of bed. Feet are not out of covers in sleep. Prefers to sleep on her abdomen (2), sprawled out (2), because it's cooler. Averse to sleeping on her back (2).

Hollow sensation in her chest (1), extends to the throat, several times a day. Very brief, as if everything stops inside. Short of breath with exertion (1): walking upstairs, lifting, and riding a bike. Constriction in throat only once. Averse to clothing around her neck, all her life (2).

Vaginal discharge, which is irritating at times.

Legs swell periodically.

Sometimes it is difficult to talk; can't find the right word (2), especially if not comfortable around someone. Will trip over her words, find another way to say what she wants. Feels foolish (2).

Desires meat (1) and butter (1). Had liked oysters (2) for a long time before she began oyster farming. Hungry a lot (2). Hunger feels like physical tension (2), then overeats (2) and eats too fast. Gained eight pounds in the past few months.

Averse to excess fat or butter (1).

Thirst is normal.

Cramp in abdomen only with great exertion. Dances hard (2) when dances, and it causes a cramp.

Physical Examination:
- Pulse: 108.
- Blood Pressure: 110/68.
- Heart: regular rate and rhythm.

(I felt that a chlamydia culture was indicated, because the discharge was unusual for her. I waited to prescribe, pending the result, which was negative.)

Phone Call: October 2, 1986

The patient called two days after her visit to tell me about her tantrums. Can be very destructive. Can't tolerate being in the other woman's presence (3). Irritated by her (3). Angry with herself (3) and takes it out on others. Hard to talk because she is so mad (3) and so frustrated inside (3). Needs some kind of outburst to release the feeling (3). Has had outbursts all her life: screaming, yelling, and throwing things. "Something physical, a release." Feels no control when it's happening. Feels better if she can be alone; then is able to calm down. Build up of pressure causes sighing.

Second Prescription and Follow-Up on Case Number 2

At this point, I believe the remedy is obvious. The extreme anger and jealousy, the need for some sort of outburst to get relief, the loquacity (present since the first visit), the intolerance of heat, the rapid heart rate, the sensitivity to clothing around her neck, the shortness of breath during exertion, the unrefreshing sleep, and the desire for oysters all point toward Lachesis. She was given one dose of Lachesis 200c. I'd like to bring your attention back to the first follow-up visit, where she reported a new symptom: a sensation of constriction or lump in her external throat. There were some hints of Lachesis in the original case, and, with the help of the Pulsatilla, we can see the case gradually evolving into a very clear Lachesis state.

Following the Lachesis, she reported improvement in several areas. She said she was more calm and relaxed. She still didn't like the "other woman," but it no longer angered her in the same way and she wasn't having tantrums about it. Her breathing was more calm and regular. She described her breath as feeling more free than in a long time. Her heart rate was still elevated, usually around 110. Her sleep was more restful. She still sprawled out in bed, although she was not over-heating as she did initially. She had only slight shortness of breath with much exertion. There was less pain and stiffness in her feet and in general.

Repertorization of the September 1986 case:

	Lach.	Kali-c.	Lyc.	Sulph.	Nat-m.	Puls.	Sep.	Apis	Nux-v.
Total	19	14	14	14	12	12	12	11	11
Rubrics	8	7	6	7	5	7	7	6	5
Generalities; AIR; open; desire for	2	1	3	3	2	3	1	2	
Mind; ANGER	1	3	3	3	3	1	3	2	3
Mind; JEALOUSY	3	2	1			2		2	2
Extremities; STIFFNESS; morning	2						1		
Extremity Pain; FOOT; sole; stepping, when				1		1			
Chest; EMPTINESS, sensation of		2		1			2		
External Throat; CLOTHING agg.	3	2					2	2	
Mind; MEMORY; weakness of; words, for	2	2	2	2	2	1			2
Respiration; DIFFICULT; exertion, after	3	2	3	2	3	2	1	2	2
Sleep; UNREFRESHING	3		2	2	2	2	2	1	2

February 11, 1987

I continued to follow her progress, and, in February 1987 (nine months after the initial visit), repeated the blood tests. Her T3 was reduced by 50 percent, and everything else was about the same. She reported feeling a little worse than at the previous visit, but overall felt her symptoms were about 25 percent of what they were originally. The symptoms that still bothered her were her heart beating hard again, swelling in the legs, shortness of breath, and feeling hot and restless at night. She also complained of eczema on her tibias, something she would often get in the winter.

I repeated the Lachesis 200c, which again seemed to help her.

April 14, 1987

The eczema on her tibias had continued since February. It first began in the winter of 1984. Has gotten progressively worse in the last few months. Itches terribly (3); aggravated by sweets (2). Voluptuous itching (3): can't avoid scratching (3); feels good to scratch because it stings, and that is a relief from the itch! Aggravated by heat in any form (2) and from thinking about it. (Very excoriated eczema; diffuse over both tibias.)

She had a bad chest cold at the end of March. Generally has been feeling very good as the cold resolved. Sweats profusely (2) since the cold, mostly on the head, axillae, hands, and feet.

She had the hollow sensation in her chest during the cold; none since becoming well. No shortness of breath. Her heart feels fairly normal.

Sleep is generally good. Occasionally it is difficult to relax. Feels rested on waking. Sleeps on her abdomen (2) and side (1). She is more comfortable on her back than she used to be. No salivation; rarely uncovers her feet.

She has been performing music lately. Played for four hours straight without difficulty! Loves to perform (2). "It's my thing!"

Emotionally, feeling better. More stable than in the past. Jealous when she sees husband talking to the other woman, but it is not extreme and passes easily. The jealousy no longer hangs on and devours her for days.

She still feels things intensely, but the feelings dissipate more easily. Tends to want things her way (2); gets so frustrated (2). Able to find a compromise after a while.

Appetite and digestion are good. Weight is stable at 155 pounds. She was really hungry today at 11 a.m., after eating a good breakfast. Hasn't had the gnawing hunger as before. Still eats quite a bit, but not excessive. Bowel movements are regular.

Desires sweets (2) and butter/oil.

Averse to oysters.

Thirsty (2) for cold drinks (1).

Warm (1).

Third Prescription and Follow-Up on Case Number 2

I am often reluctant to change the prescription when someone is improving. I felt particularly reluctant in this case because the symptoms seemed to be focusing on the skin. Nevertheless, the patient was truly suffering from her eczema and had already tried palliative topical treatments (baking soda, colloidal oatmeal, chamomile) without relief. It was very clear to me that if I didn't help her, she would resort to more drastic and, perhaps, disruptive measures. It was also very clear to me that she needed Sulphur.

Repertorization of the April 1987 case:

	Sulph.	Lyc.	Merc.	Puls.	Sep.	Ars.	Petr.	Nat-m.	Rhus-t.
Total	17	14	12	11	11	8	8	8	8
Rubrics	7	6	6	6	5	4	4	4	4
Extremities; ERUPTION; Leg; eczema	3	2	2			3	3	2	2
Skin; ERUPTIONS; itching; warmth; agg.	2	2	3	2					
Skin; ITCHING; scratch; until it is raw	2	2	1	1	2		3		2
Skin; ITCHING; voluptuous	3		2	1	1				
Perspiration; PROFUSE	2	3	3	2	3	3	1	3	2
Sleep; POSITION; abdomen, on	2	2		3	3	1		2	
Stomach; DESIRES; sweets	3	3	1	2	2	1	1	1	2

So, I gave her one dose of Sulphur 200c. This prescription was based on the following: her eruption, which was worse from warmth; itching, which was voluptuous; scratching until the eruption was raw and bleeding; profuse perspiration; and her description of her love of performance and the need for an audience—something she had apparently felt a lot in her life but her own vital energy had no need to bring it out prior to this time.

May 1987

She came back in six weeks (12 months after initial visit) and again reported improvement:

Her legs were almost completely cleared, after getting even worse in the first week after the remedy.

She has had no hollow sensation in her chest; this has been gone for a long time. She sometimes feels her heart beating fast, but it is not routine. She is a little short of breath on exertion, but it feels more like it is resulting from being out of shape rather than from having something wrong with her. She hasn't noticed any side cramps. These have gradually decreased since the beginning of her treatment.

She reports a whole change in attitude. A year ago she was feeling very weak, lacking energy, helpless and angry, and not productive or creative. She now says she has much more of a perspective on things. She is really happy with her current lifestyle and feels energetic.

Her pulse at this visit was 80. She says it has generally been about 80 when she has checked it periodically over the last number of weeks.

Her next visit was three months later.

September 22, 1987

This visit was 16 months after the initial visit.

She was feeling tired the last couple of months.

Low energy, depressed.

Feeling uncomfortable around people (2); wants to hide (2).

Physically feels run down (2) and heavy (2). Has energy for working, and is able to do it, but feels incompetent (3), clumsy (2), and down on self (2).

Sleeping well. Rested on waking, but tired again within one hour. No need for naps.

Occasional hollow sensation in chest; occasional rapid heart. Generally has been feeling okay. Pulse averages 90 to 95.

Feels tense (2), not at ease (2), like holding her breath in, then sighs (2).

(Much sighing throughout interview.)

(Tears.) Wants someone else to make her feel good and take care of her. Doesn't feel she has the ability to feel great. Mildly depressed most of her life. Lives from one performance to the next, like a binge; depression (2) returns when a performance is over. Wants to eat when depressed (2), and be alone (1). Feels muddle-headed, stupid, and uninformed (2). Sits around thinking about her life and her depression (2). Unable to make decisions (2).

Menses June 15 and July 9. Menses in July began with one week of dark brown mucus-like discharge, spotting, then flow for one week. Stopped one week, then bled again for a week. This has never happened before. Menses on August 31 was normal.

Desires sweets (2) and salt (1).

Averse to yams (2) and marshmallows (2).

Thirstless.

Sleeps on her abdomen (2) with windows open (2). Feet stay covered; no salivation.

Desires open air (3).

Fourth Prescription and Follow-Up on Case Number 2

There is a distinct progression of symptoms in the case. Her hyperthyroid symptoms are virtually resolved. She notices an occasional rapid heart rate, but the heat and agitation and the trembling and weakness that originally accompanied her condition have been absent for quite some time. She seems to be getting down to the "essence" of the problems that plagued her from childhood: a great lack of confidence, a feeling of being forsaken, reproaching herself, and being irresolute and introspective. These symptoms, along with the desire for open air, an intermittent menses, and her thirstlessness led me to once again give her Pulsatilla, one dose of 1M.

Repertorization of the September 1987 case:

	Puls.	Aur.	Ign.	Sulph.	Lach.	Lyc.	Alum.	Nat-m.	Stram.
Total	23	15	15	15	14	13	12	12	11
Rubrics	10	7	7	8	7	7	8	7	6
Mind; CONFIDENCE want of self	2	2	1	1	1	2	1	1	1
Mind; FORSAKEN feeling	3	3			2		1		2
Mind; REPROACHES; himself	2	2	2			1		2	
Mind; SIGHING	1		3	1	1		1	1	2
Mind; INTROSPECTION	3	2	3	2			1		
Mind; IRRESOLUTION	2	1	3	2	3	2	2	2	
Generalities; LASSITUDE	1	2	2	2	3	2	3	2	2
Female Genitalia; MENSES; intermittent	3			2	2	1	1		
Sleep; POSITION; abdomen, on	3		1	2		2		2	2
Generalities; AIR; open; desire for	3	3		3	2	3	2	2	2

April 1988

I didn't see her again until the following April (23 months after the initial visit). She reported dramatic changes in the last six months:

Her energy has been very good for many months. She is really loving her work and says that life is a joy! In January, she started nude modeling for an art class and was really enjoying it. Her improved self-image is allowing her to do it, and doing it further improves her self-image. She has started giving piano lessons, something she has always lacked confidence to do. Her periods have been regular and pain-free. Her pulse has generally been around 80. She has not noticed any hyperthyroid symptoms.

She didn't remember having taken a remedy six months earlier. When I read to her from the previous case, she was shocked to be reminded of how bad she had felt, because she hadn't felt that way for so long.

Lab tests at the end of March showed her T3 to be 196 (normal = 85-185). All other tests were well within the normal limits.

September 20, 1988

She came in complaining that her "brain was not functioning well." She felt dull-brained. She couldn't put words together, think of words, or remember things such as names. She had difficulty comprehending what she read, "even a menu," and was feeling overwhelmed by it. She felt dumb. It had been gradually building up since her last office visit. (You might recall that she described a little bit of this at her second visit, 2 1/2 years earlier, but it hadn't become the focus of the case until now. Clearly she is working her way back through many years and layers of pathology.)

She felt this way after she first smoked marijuana a few times. She felt that something was damaged. This has gotten much worse in the last few months. She is depressed and feels down on herself. She feels that everyone else is witty and bright and that she is stupid. No one around her notices her difficulty or is aware of how she is feeling. Her life is going fairly well, but she is preoccupied with feeling fat and stupid.

Her sleep is disturbed, waking in the night and being awake for several hours. She is very tired during the day and tries to nap, but can't sleep.

She is very constipated, with a lot of gas. She is strongly craving bread, sweets, beer and alcohol every night.

Physically, she is feeling well. She has not had any return of her original symptoms.

She is avoiding her relatives because she doesn't want to deal with appearing stupid. She is only interested in sleeping, eating, and sex. Her sex desire continues to be strong.

She says that she "can't help but feel that the current problems all go back a long time, pretty deep and old."

Fifth Prescription and Follow-Up on Case Number 2

I gave her one dose of Lycopodium 200c. This prescription was based on the information she gave me, particularly on the following three symptoms: her apparent ability to function in company so that no one knew she was feeling stupid and having difficulty with her mind (to function behind a façade), the complaints of constipation and gas, and the desire for alcohol.

Repertorization of the September 1988 case:

	Lyc.	Nat-m.	Nux-v.	Puls.	Sulph.	Am-c.	Ars.	Bry.	Chin.
Total	19	16	17	19	20	9	13	14	15
Rubrics	8	8	8	8	8	7	7	7	7
Mind; DULLNESS	3	3	2	3	3	1	1	3	2
Mind; FORGETFUL; words, of, while speaking	2	2	2		1				
Sleep; WAKING; frequent	2	2	2	3	3	1	2	2	2
Rectum; CONSTIPATION; difficult stool	2	3	3	2	3	2		3	1
Rectum; FLATUS	3	2	3	3	3		2	2	3
Stomach; THIRSTLESS	2	1	1	3	1	1	2	1	3
Stomach; DESIRES; bread		2		1		1	2		
Stomach; DESIRES; alcoholic drinks	2		3	2	3	1	3	1	1
Stomach; DESIRES; sweets	3	1	1	2	3	2	1	2	3

November 1988

Six weeks later she reported great improvement. Her feeling of withdrawal had really lightened up. She was no longer feeling bad or stupid. She occasionally has difficulty finding words, but rarely. "I have a sense of calm." She started feeling better almost immediately after the remedy, on the way home. She can't really remember feeling bad since her last office visit.

She really wants to lose weight. Her appetite is less. She isn't preoccupied with food, but gets overwhelmed with the preparation of food. She has lost her craving for sweets. She still craves alcohol, though this craving is less.

There is still some constipation, but less. She continued to have a problem with gas for a while, but that is better now. She is sleeping well, and physically feeling good. She feels that she is on to the next thing, an old problem, more subtle — a feeling that there are certain things in herself that she would like to change. She wants something to make her feel perfect.

September 25, 1989

The next time I saw her was a year later (three years, four months from her initial visit).

She said that she had generally been feeling good. She has had recurrent yeast vaginitis through the year and has mostly treated it with boric acid and acidophilus. She has not used anything for the last six to eight months, and the symptoms seem to come and go.

She has been very constipated, with a small, sticky stool; it is not hard, but she strains to pass it. Her intestines feel clogged up.

She is concerned about her mental state. She gets very spaced out. It becomes hard to talk in certain situations, such as when she has to make choices or express abstract thought. It is difficult to think of the words and causes her to feel stupid; it is like a foggy cloud over her head.

Her eyes feel gravelly. She believes her eyeballs got larger from the hyperthyroid and have remained so. (Her eyes appear normal to me, and an ophthalmologic examination confirms that they are normal.) She feels that her whole head has become bigger, including her throat and tongue. She feels that her tongue is so large that it fills her mouth.

Her appetite is reduced, and she has lost some weight. She is craving potato chips.

Her sleep is good, but lately she is waking early, around 4 a.m.

Sixth Prescription and Follow-Up on Case Number 2

Alumina has the characteristic of constipation, with a soft stool. Alumina patients can have the delusion that body parts are enlarged, can have acrid leucorrhea, and they can make mistakes in speaking. They have a particular kind of mental confusion, a dull slowness of comprehension making it difficult for them to get their thoughts and feelings out; there is both a physical and a mental constipation. They can either crave or be averse to potatoes.

She was given one dose of Alumina 200c, after which she reported that her eyes were less dry and itchy. There was still some gravelly sensation, but much less, and it would resolve by mid-day. Her head still felt large, but it was very subtle. Her tongue no longer felt large. Her bowels were better. She was having regular bowel movements without difficulty. She felt cleansed after a bowel movement rather than clogged up; this change occurred immediately after the remedy.

She still has some difficulty finding words when speaking, mostly descriptive words, but she hasn't been feeling spacy for quite some time. She no longer has the sensation of a fog descending. Her mood has generally been good. She notices herself feeling less intruded on by others and is gradually feeling more and more open to people she would previously have been closed to.

Repertorization of the September 1989 case:

	Alum.	Nat-m.	Puls.	Sep.	Sulph.	Zinc.	Lyc.	Sil.
Total	17	15	15	13	11	10	11	9
Rubrics	8	7	6	6	6	6	5	6
Female Genitalia; LEUCORRHOEA; white	2	3	2	3	1	2		1
Female Genitalia; LEUCORRHOEA; acrid,...	3	2	3	3	2	1	3	3
Rectum; CONSTIPATION; difficult stool; soft stool	3	2	2	3	1	1	1	2
Mind; MISTAKES; speaking	2	3	2	1	1	1	2	1
Mind; CONFUSION; talking, while		2						
Mind; DELUSIONS; large; parts of body seem too	1							
Stomach; DESIRES; potatoes	1							
Eye; DRYNESS	3	1	3	2	3	3	3	1
Eye; ITCHING	2	2	3	1	3	2	2	1

Summary of Prescriptions

Date	Remedy	Time From Last Remedy
5/12/86	Pulsatilla 200c	
9/30/86	Lachesis 200c	4 1/2 months
2/11/87	Lachesis 200c	4 1/2 months
4/14/87	Sulphur 200c	2 months
9/22/87	Pulsatilla 1M	5 1/2 months
9/20/88	Lycopodium 200c	1 year
9/25/89	Alumina 200c	1 year

Conclusion for Case Number 2

This case is noteworthy for several reasons. The first item of note is the results of the blood tests. The thyroid levels didn't come down into the normal range until March/April 1988, two years after her treatment began, even though her hyperthyroid symptoms were significantly reduced within the first few months of treatment. It is also of note that, *after* she began having improvement of her symptoms, her liver enzymes and glucose levels were elevated. An aggravation perhaps?

In addition, the evolution of the case provides a good example of Hering's Law. Although homeopaths often refer to Hering's Law in talking about healing taking place in the reverse order of appearance of symptoms, I think it is rather rare to actually get to see this phenomenon played out so graphically. It is also unusual to see the evolution into deeper layers come through so clearly in terms of symptoms pointing to the next prescription.

This woman came in complaining of hyperthyroidism, of a few months' duration. Pulsatilla began the process of healing. Initially, there were hints of Lachesis, hints of Lycopodium and Sulphur, and hints of Alumina. Lachesis was brought out more strongly, I believe, by the Pulsatilla (after which she began noticing a constriction in her throat) and by her circumstances: the suppression of her feelings and herself in her relationship and the lack of an emotional outlet.

Following this, her eczema of two years' duration became the worst it had ever been. Sulphur moved her through this layer. I have a tendency to think that once the patient gets to the level of terrible skin eruptions, it should be the end of the case. But, for this woman, it was just the beginning.

It was as if all of the remedies to this point were stripping away recent layers so that she could get back to the significant emotional pathology that had plagued her during her younger years. This stripping away brought her back to the Pulsatilla state: the lost and neglected little girl who ate excessively to "fill" herself up. And, from this state, she gradually, over the next year, began confronting more directly her confidence issues, which were helped by Lycopodium.

After this, the case took an interesting twist. It moved into the Alumina state, which was hinted at in the original case (constipation all her life, before hyperthyroid). I find myself wondering if the lack of confidence didn't, at least in part, develop out of a mental weakness that existed from a very early age.

Finally, I would like to make a point regarding the amount of time between prescriptions. The first few remedies prescribed were given an average of four or five months apart, and the last few were one year apart. This makes sense in light of how long she had been suffering from each of the various conditions. We have a general idea that it takes one month of healing for every year that the person has been sick. I can't say that I have ever observed this to be precisely true, but it makes sense to me that the layers relating to her mental and emotional struggles originating in her childhood would be "thicker" and that the remedies would act for longer periods of time without changing image.

Warren Metzler: My experience with Pulsatilla patients is that they are rather weak internally. As a result, they want someone else to set up a structure for them, but then they want to run the structure once they are in it. In this case, I believe if you had given Pulsatilla 1M when you gave Lachesis 200c, it would not have been necessary to give Lachesis and Sulphur. I have learned over the years never to leave a remedy before its action is completely finished.

Kipnis: An interesting point. One can only wonder what might have happened in this case if that had been done.

Herb Joiner-Bey: Something I learned from Dr. Robin Murphy is to use Arsenicum iodatum for the severe night sweats in AIDS patients. The remedy has worked well for me in the acute context.

Kipnis: Just for night sweats, not touching the other levels of the disease?

Herb Joiner-Bey: It does not seem to affect the other aspects. It mainly acts to reduce the night sweats, and then other remedies are needed.

Jeff Baker, ND, DHANP

A REMEDY
PRESCRIBED
BY A KEYNOTE
REVEALS ITS TOTALITY
& ESSENCE

Jeff Baker, ND, DHANP, is a graduate of the National College of Naturopathic Medicine. He also is a 1983 graduate of the IFH Professional Course, studied with George Vithoulkas from 1984 to 1986, and is a diplomate of the Homeopathic Academy of Naturopathic Physicians. After seven years of busy practice in Northern California, Jeff recently moved to Maui, Hawaii, where he is building his practice and a new home simultaneously, while raising three children. After 10 years of "Fifth Organon prescribing," he is now actively investigating Hahnemann's "Sixth Organon posology" and intends to share his findings in 1991.

Introduction

This is exciting for me. Although I can't lay claim to being from a long line of homeopaths, I can say with great sincerity that my family really lives, breathes, and sleeps homeopathy. In fact, the night before I left Maui for Seattle my three-year-old son cried out in his sleep, "I can't get my remedy bottle open." Then he went back to sleep. So sweet.

It occurred to me that this whole business of "small remedies" surely has to have a humorous side in the eyes of our allopathic brethren. As if our dosages had anything tangible in them in the first place and then we have the audacity to call a whole class of our medicines "small remedies." In that vein, I'm both pleased and honored to present a homeopathic sequel to *The Emperor's New Clothes*.

The science of homeopathy is composed of a body of knowledge that is not static, but rather is ever expanding. From time to time each of us is given the rare opportunity to contribute to homeopathy's dynamic organism. This presentation is about just such an opportunity — the in vivo evolution of a remedy. It is a thought-provoking and fascinating process that leaves one in awe of homeopathy's progenitors and great masters, without whose perceptiveness and vast contributions we'd be lost. We owe an undying debt of gratitude to all of them. I'd like to single out George Vithoulkas, who, as you will see, was instrumental in making this paper possible.

There's an old adage that we've all heard, "The proof of the pudding is in the eating." I believe Dr. Hahnemann must have subscribed to this notion, because he proved 89 remedies in his lifetime. Most of us resort to these and other well-proven remedies for the majority of our cases. Indeed, throughout the history of homeopathy, many astute practitioners have recommended that, for the most part, we stick close to the well-proven remedies — remedies whose physical, mental, and emotional patho-logical states are fairly well-delineated in the materia medicas. We can confirm our prescriptions of these remedies in a fairly straightforward fashion and, if the symp-toms seem to fit, prescribe with some degree of confidence.

But what about all the remedies that haven't been well proven or even proven at all? Surely they must have their own distinctive pictures and uses. What about all those cases that don't quite progress the way we'd like them to? I have my share of skeletons in the closet. And I believe any sincere, honest homeopath could probably make that statement. One of the cures for this disease of homeopathic ignorance is possession of an ever-expanding scope of materia medica.

This paper is about a remedy that has not been proven and therefore is much less likely to be given. Additionally, its drug picture, vis-a-vis materia medica, is rather linear and is limited to a narrow scope of physical complaints. How I've been able to glean the picture of such a remedy is the first part of the story.

It begins in 1986, when a female patient of mine was suffering with an infected boil. George Vithoulkas was teaching in Berkeley at the time, and I was fortunate to be able to arrange for him to see her at the seminar. I was at a loss as to what to do. I thought it would be an interesting and perhaps instructive little case but had no idea of where it would lead.

I am presenting this case and two other cases. Each of the three cases has revealed to me the totality and essence of this particular remedy, and each has no less than two years of follow-up. I will also briefly describe one other case that shared similar physical symptoms with the first three cases but did not manifest the same emotional qualities.

Case Number 1

Female, Age 38

I know that some of you are familiar with this case. Please be so kind as not to divulge the remedy so that the rest of the participants can have an opportunity to read and think through the case on their own. For those of you who know the remedy and may even have heard or read the earlier presentation I gave three years ago at the HANP conference, I'd like to say that the information in the earlier presentation was premature and incomplete. It reflected my limited understanding up to that point.

What I have to share with you today is, I believe, much more cohesive and therefore of potentially much greater use to the community of practicing homeopaths.

October 1986

This woman had a very large boil on the back of the right clavicle. It was 3 x 6 centimeters across and about 5 centimeters deep (3), very invasive (3), and extremely inflamed (4). She described a burning heat. She said the word "burning" didn't do justice to the amount of pain she was experiencing, and alternately she spoke of a "searing" sensation. There was a deep reddish discoloration, and unremitting excruciating pain. It was very hot to the touch (3) and indurated (3). She hadn't been able to sleep for the past two nights.

Previously, this lesion was a cyst that had existed for eight years — an innocuous golf-ball-sized sebaceous cyst with no pain or sensation. One week ago it began to discharge. It had briefly discharged once about five years earlier. She was now pregnant and at the conclusion of her second trimester. When this recent discharge began, her husband manually expressed it. Over the next two to three days, three tablespoons of thick white discharge came out. It smelled like strong cheese. During this same period, her mental and emotional states were breaking down, and she was becoming physically exhausted.

On the fourth day of this episode, she was given a dose of Pulsatilla lM on the basis of certain strong characteristics and the fact that she had reacted well to it in the past. The following indications were present: great weepiness, extremely emotional, drained of energy, wanting to be outside without any clothes on although it was fairly chilly, and quite thirstless. Within an hour after the Pulsatilla, she was much better, experiencing a remarkably positive change. Her physical energy came back, and the boil completely stopped discharging. From that point on, she did much better emotionally and her energy was much better. But, over the next four days, the boil became a malignant type of ulcer. By the time she arrived in Berkeley to see Vithoulkas, the pain was so great it totally deprived her of sleep. The lesion looked like a carbuncle, yet was unripe for incision and drainage.

Analysis of Case Number 1

I'd like to give you George Vithoulkas's analysis of the case. First, he preferred not to give any remedy because the Pulsatilla had acted so well. He said that he would have opted for some kind of surgical intervention to allow for drainage, but it was not yet the right time. He reluctantly decided to prescribe a remedy because of the degree of her suffering and because the pain was completely interfering with her sleep.

For George, the choice of remedies seemed relatively clear. There were three possibilities: Hepar sulphuris calcareum, Tarentula cubensis, and Anthracinum. Hepar was suggested because of the cheesy smelling discharge. But it was ruled out because she wasn't sensitive to touch, and she was hot. George allowed that Tarentula definitely had boils, which could burn like the one in this case, but that Tarentula lesions are more superficial and do not invade so deeply into the underlying tissue. This, he said, was the main differentiating aspect of the case.

I had been thinking of Arsenicum and Hepar but was dissatisfied by either choice. In fact, the materia medicas say that Anthracinum is indicated in boils, with great burning, when Arsenicum fails. So, Anthracinum was chosen. Boericke says of Anthracinum: "In boils and boil-like eruptions; terrible drainage; carbuncles, malignant ulcers; induration of tissue and inflammation of connective tissue where there is a purulent focus. Intolerable burning."

Plan: George instructed that she be given Anthracinum 30c, but 200c was the only potency available in the Hahnemann Pharmacy. So, a single dose of 200c was given.

Follow-Up on Case Number 1

After taking the remedy, she went to a nearby park where she sat and felt relaxed for the first time in days. The pain was relatively unchanged, but, for the first time, she felt okay about it. Over the first couple of days, the pain definitely decreased, but the carbuncle itself became enormous. George predicted that it would drain for at least a month and maybe up to a year, but he felt that Anthracinum was only a local remedy and not a deep-acting one. So, the lesion got larger, but she felt better. After about a week, it began to drain. Every time water got on it, even a drop, it would open and drain. It drained for about six weeks.

It is extremely interesting that, in the second week after the remedy, she wept almost continuously, and that the weeping was centered on a grief she had experienced 18 years earlier, when her marriage with her first husband broke up. It was a tremendous purging of emotion that had never before emerged. This woman had been given Natrum muriaticum six years earlier, and, although it had acted, the effect was minimal.

As the feelings of grief resolved, she found herself changing. Here are some notes she made at the time:

I don't even know if you could imagine what it's like to have your whole life turned upside down. The biggest thing is that I no longer have to control everything. I don't have to be the one controlling. What it's like is like being in the passenger's seat, not the driver's. I'm not in control. An enormous weight is off my shoulders, which is funny because now the bump's off my shoulder.

I have a lot of thoughts. I was always a happy person; now I'm exuberant! (Remember this statement. There is an almost identical quote in an upcoming case.) I'm more outgoing; definitely, I'm more outgoing to strangers and more spontaneous. Without even thinking, I take care of things that I would have dragged my heels with before, and now at the first opportunity I act; I don't procrastinate."

I'm more open and loving on all levels. With my eight-year-old daughter, whom I've always loved dearly but not so expressively since the last child came four years ago, now I'm openly and physically affectionate. And it's clear that she knows it, without even consciously knowing, because she reciprocates expressively, where before she was as aloof as I.

Sexually, I'm as excited and interested and active as I was before the grief happened 18 years ago. It's a state I haven't known for the last half of my life, since I was first sexually active, and obviously a state I'd enjoyed for only a brief time leading up to the grief.

Before, I took on things that were unreasonable and didn't appreciate their unreasonableness, just as I didn't know I was seeking to be in control. Now I'm able to say "no" and feel fine, where before I was indecisive, "wishy-washy."

I've experienced two emotionally heart-wrenching crying episodes (during the ten days of almost constant weeping). In both instances I awoke from sleep, the first time at 4 a.m., and the second at 1 a.m.; the first one lasted 2 1/2 hours, and the second for only one hour. The first one felt like my heart hurt so much it was going to break, and I cried and prayed the whole time. At the conclusion of the first episode, it was a relief to go back to sleep. In the second episode, I was reproaching myself for having feelings of jealousy and suspicion about my husband, but after crying for an hour it felt like I'd lost them permanently. I've felt great since then.

There's no more attachment to my first husband. There's nothing left there, not the self-reproach, nothing. It's a void, like nothing was ever there.

Vithoulkas was astounded when he heard about the deep reaction to Anthracinum early on. I felt that, with these crying episodes and the tremendous state of emotional fragility, Pulsatilla was going to be needed again, but he cautioned me to wait. He thought that Anthracinum was going extremely deep. Additionally, he thought that she had some sort of a malabsorption problem and that after she went through the pregnancy she would be in an entirely different and improved state of health and wouldn't revert back. She weighed 95 pounds before the pregnancy. He felt that something wasn't quite right in her system. Previously, she needed to eat constantly, even getting up in the middle of the night to do so. After Anthracinum, her eating became much more balanced. She was eating only regular meals; she did not crave sweets very much, which before had been very strong; and she was no longer eating before going to bed in order to make it through the night.

An old symptom returned about ten days after the remedy was given: a dry, cracking dermatitis, along with itching and bleeding. It cleared up spontaneously after only a few days. About 2 1/2 years earlier, for the first time in her life, she had developed a similar but much more severe case of cracking, bleeding dermatitis on her fingers, which had persisted for several months.

Two other notable changes occurred. A peculiar cough, a kind of paroxysmal dry, tickling cough that would send her into spasms, went away. She had this cough all her life, and her mother and maternal grandmother also suffered from it. To her, this relief was very impressive. In fact, she was rather amazed by it. The other change was that she didn't need to urinate during the night through the rest of the pregnancy. She had never been free of this with her prior two pregnancies.

She has continued to do very well. Over the past 3 1/2 years, her general health has improved appreciably. Before Anthracinum, her general health was adversely affected by certain environmental exposures: strong odors; petroleum-based products, such as gasoline and pesticides; or just exposure to new fabric in a fabric or a clothing store. Any of these exposures could bring on anorexia, nausea, weight loss, motion sickness, or dermatitis on her hands. These symptoms are reminiscent of a Petroleum picture, which indeed is one of the remedies she had once needed. Now, none of these exposures seem to have any particular effect on her.

Another problem she had was a great fear at night when her husband was away. She would barricade herself and the children in a room with the telephone as soon as it would become dark. In 1983, she was given Medorrhinum, which partially helped this phobia. Since Anthracinum, this is no longer an issue for her.

She still tends to be somewhat of a workaholic and desires salt and sweets. She has taken Calcarea carbonica, with benefit, twice in the past two years. Her energy is abundant, she's gained some weight, and is not as prone to becoming so thin and gaunt. She's a little more chilly than she used to be, but basically she's asymptomatic. Even the coughing problem is relatively quiescent. What remains of the cyst is a pea-sized lump, where previously there was a tumor the size of a golf ball.

I'd like to mention one last point in relation to carbuncles and Anthracinum. The following is a footnote from the Anthracinum section in Hering's Guiding Symptoms: "To call a carbuncle a surgical case is the greatest absurdity. An incision is always injurious and often the cause of death. Never a case has been lost under the right kind of treatment, and carbuncles should always be treated by internal medicine only."

Case Number 2

Female, Age 26

Initial Interview: December 29, 1986

Chief Complaint: eczema (2)
- Dorsum of fingers (2); cracks and itches (2). It is also on her face, above the eyebrows.
- Fluid-filled vesicles; worse from pinching, which makes the watery fluid exude (1).
- She has had the eczema on her hands since her marriage (six years ago), but on other areas since birth. As an infant, she had eruptions behind her knees that would exude after waking from sleep and extending the legs.
- There are little circular patches (2) on her arms and legs (1), which itch less than her fingers; the patches can be somewhat reddened.
- The itching is worse at night (2); wakes her from a sound sleep (2).
- The eczema is better in the summer (3), from the sun; as soon as the sun comes up, she's out in it "because it's healing."
- It is worse in the winter (2), from wind, dryness, and dry indoor heat (2).

She has hay fever, which "comes and goes." The main symptoms are sneezing (2) and watery eyes "a little." She doesn't have it every year. When she was younger, she had it four years in a row.

Presumptive diagnosis of gonorrhea at age 17 because her boyfriend had it. She had two yeast infections around the same age. They may have been due to birth control pills, which she took for two or three years. "Messed me up by having menstrual cycles every two or three weeks."

She has a "pinched nerve" in her right hip (1). It is a familial problem; her mother and maternal grandmother also have it. It is worse from bending or carrying and immediately better following reflexology.

She suffered from motion sickness up to age seven; nausea, but no vomiting.

She has had cysts "all the time" (2). Years ago, she had one on her left cheek that went away and left a palpable induration. She had another on her right forehead at age 17 or 18, one on her left temple one year ago that just recently went away, and two different cysts on her external vagina in the last year, which erupted premenstrually and abated by themselves.

In the last one to two years, she has been "tense and impatient," starting about two weeks before menses and lasting until the onset (1). She is better with the onset (2), "the day it starts." In the last year, she also has had tender breasts (1) during this two-week period. They are sore to touch or from a bump. She yells at her children, from irritability (1). One time last spring, it was so bad that she thought she was going crazy.

Her menses are regular. She feels her very best after her menses are over, and she doesn't feel bad during menses (no cramps or other discomforts).

She has had two pregnancies, two births, and no abortions. Her two children are boys, ages five and three.

Desires sweets (3), seasoned (2) Mexican food, chicken (1), orange juice (1), chocolate (3), and butter (1).

Averse to "fishy taste" (2) and fat of meat (3), even skin of chicken. Indifferent to fruit. Wipes excess salt off chips. "Eggs must be cooked just right or they sicken me."

Normal thirst, for cold drinks (1).

Her eyes have been sensitive to the sun (1) in the last year.

Averse to warm, stuffy environments (2) but keeps the windows closed at night because of her fear; opens them in the summer only if it is really hot.

Is afraid of being alone in the house at night, even with her boys. This fear of being alone at night (2) was there even before she had children.

She also has a strong fear of her husband dying in a car accident (3). "If he's 15 minutes late I have him dead and buried in my mind, with a funeral."

She is nervous when her husband is driving the family in foggy or wet conditions or in lots of traffic (2). "Not if I'm driving because then I'm in control."

She is sensitive (2) and sympathetic (1); mostly even-tempered and in a good mood. Occasionally she is sad, with depressed feelings. She usually is more moody around her menses and feels sorry for herself.

Is a good sleeper; goes right to sleep; the first five minutes of waking are difficult (1). Sleeps on her back or left side (1); the right side is not as comfortable (1). Before having children, she slept on her abdomen only.

Her hands and feet are always cold (3). She is chilly in general (1).

Her eczema is better with something cold on it (1). For example, the itching is better when she puts her hands on cool sheets, her cold hands on the facial eruption, or her feet out of the covers.

She perspires in her axillae when she is nervous (1).

Digestion and elimination are good; daily bowel movements.

Rare to have headaches.

Averse to being alone (1); likes to be with people (2).

She likes consolation, but doesn't seek it out.

Doesn't cry often, but can when she is alone (l).

Her sex drive is normal; twice a week is good for her.

She has been married for seven years; it is a good marriage.

Her father died in a car accident when she was seven years old. "I didn't let it affect me." She forgot everything about him very shortly afterwards. Six months ago, she began crying when thinking about him; lasted for one month.

Need for control (l).

Her grandfather died eight months ago. She cried a bit; tries to hold it in until she is alone.

She was always afraid to show emotions because she did not want to be hurt (2). Always felt vulnerable, so she avoided showing emotions.

Was very hurt from her mother's drinking all through the patient's high school years.

Analysis of Case Number 2

This was the first time the patient had sought homeopathic treatment. As the case unfolded, I thought mostly about Natrum muriaticum, Petroleum, and Sulphur. But something about each of these choices just didn't satisfy me.

The history of grief and the totality of symptoms, including hay fever, premenstrual tension, and sleep position, fit Natrum muriaticum. But the strong amelioration of the eczema in the sun was not easily reconcilable. Also, her chilliness and food desires didn't fit very well.

Petroleum was an idea that I probed, and, if the case had presented one more strong confirmation, I might have given it. I would like to have seen not only a history of motion sickness up to age seven, as she reported, but also something more current in that regard. Or, if she had sensitivities to petroleum products, I would have taken that as a clue. But neither of these was present. Moreover, the mental and emotional components of the case were fairly strong. Although it took a certain amount of probing to bring these aspects of the case out, once revealed, I felt they could not be ignored.

Regarding the idea of Sulphur, I just wasn't able to convince myself to bend this into a Sulphur case. Again, some of the data fit — the eczema, the food desires, the anxiety about her husband, and the sleep position — but something about her did not resonate with my experience of Sulphur.

Actually, as I was taking this woman's case, something about her and the way she presented herself led me to think of my first Anthracinum patient. They were very similar in terms of body type and demeanor. They both possessed a soft, sweet nature in addition to a lack of assertiveness.

I noticed in thumbing through the repertory that Anthracinum is listed for cracking dermatitis of the fingers (italics). This led me to ask the patient about cysts, which she definitely confirmed. About 90 to 95 percent of the time, I prescribe at the time of the visit, but, although I wanted to give Anthracinum right then, something made me hesitate. The intuitive part of me said "yes," but my practical, intellectual side rebelled. So, I took the case home and leafed through it every couple of days for about a week. Finally, I said to myself, "What the heck! It'll most likely either do nothing or maybe it'll produce a miracle."

Plan: I gave Anthracinum 200c, a single dose.

Follow-Up on Case Number 2

First Follow-Up: February 24, 1987

"I'm just fine."

The itching (l) has markedly decreased. She is not waking up at night from the itching, and it's winter, which is usually the worst time.

For the most part, the fluid-filled bumps are gone.

Her skin is really dry in the eczematous areas (2).

She wasn't on edge the two weeks before her menses; only the night before her menses and as it began. Didn't crave chocolate. Her appetite increased, but only one day before her menses instead of the whole two weeks before.

Other symptoms that were not mentioned in the original case:

She clenches and grinds her teeth at night (1), especially "with worry and at times of stress." Her husband has heard her grind her teeth in her sleep in the past.

Has had tonsillitis for the last five years; she's had it on and off all her life; as a child, she took antibiotics; remembers the problem since age 12 and recalls taking antibiotics about once each winter.

Itching from handling wet cat fur (2).

(The two symptoms, the teeth grinding in sleep and the recurrent tonsillitis, make us think of Tuberculinum.)

Back to the follow-up:

Her hip is much better.

The craving for sweets and chocolate (1) has decreased.

Ten days after taking the remedy, she got really sick with a "flu." She was so exhausted she couldn't get up for seven days; just slept constantly. She had never been so sick; mostly, it was just exhaustion. Strangely enough, she had a big appetite throughout.

(When I asked her to enumerate the symptoms of this so-called flu, she had none to relate. Simply, she had been plunged into a state where all she could do for one whole week was sleep. Vithoulkas has emphasized that this is the best response you can get after a remedy and that the patient must go to bed and take all the sleep that is required. In this situation, all the portals of energy expenditure are closed off in order to allow the vital force to focus entirely on healing. I pointed out to her that this really was not a flu because she had no fever, chills, muscle aches, or nausea. She agreed. It's essential that we tell our patients that they must abide by what their organism is telling them, because, if they fight against it, they will blunt the action of the remedy.)

Her hands and feet are less cold. Her feet are cold at night in bed between 3 and 5 a.m. (2); this wakes her up.

Finds herself telling her husband things she wouldn't have before; this surprises her because she wouldn't have done this in the past for fear of being hurt.

Two days after taking the remedy, she went through a period when she cried a lot about her father. "Wish I had my daddy. Such a strange thought because I never had that thought before, even though I had thought about him a lot." Even now, she could easily come to tears thinking about him. Sharing all this with her husband has forged a stronger bond.

Sex is more enjoyable, and there is more closeness with her husband. Her sex drive has increased; she is more open and free.

Assessment: A remarkable and positive response to Anthracinum.

Plan: No remedy. Return to clinic in two months.

Second Follow-Up: April 28, 1987

Her energy is a lot better.

There is a definite letting down of all barriers; she feels they were there because of the possibility of something happening to her husband similar to what happened to her father, and not wanting to be hurt. She is able to get even closer to her husband; "able to admit to failure" with husband.

"Always felt like I was a happy person but feel much happier, more relaxed." (Here's that very same remark again. I'll refer to it when I tie the common threads together.)

The bumps of fluid are gone, but her skin is dry (2), cracked (1), and gradually becoming itchier (2).

The sun feels so good on her skin (3) but without the usual amelioration.

Lots more cysts (2) around the face (2) and vaginal area (1) (external labia). No burning sensations. They occur randomly, not before menses, as before.

Her last menses came on a 23-day interval and lasted one day longer than usual (five days). Her water retention lasted one week after the menses, mostly in her abdomen (2) and thighs. She usually "feels fat" only until the menses. She then urinated frequently for two days, and it went away.

Desires sweets (1 1/2); not particularly for chocolate as before.

Was on edge before her menses, but it was still better than originally.

Driving with her husband is easier, less anxiety provoking. She is not completely better, but not nearly as nervous.

Her husband hasn't been gone, so her fear of being alone and her anxiety about him remain untested.

Some sneezing (1) from seasonal pollens.

Her ability to be intimate with her husband is "a lot, a lot" better, and sex is so much more enjoyable. (Rendered spontaneously at the conclusion of the interview.)

Assessment: She is doing fabulously well.

Plan: No remedy. Return to the clinic in four months.

Later Follow-Ups

On subsequent follow-ups she reported that she felt resolved and at peace in her relationship to her dad. Interestingly, she experienced some grief about having to give her dog away. She said she cried and cried and didn't want to do it. She didn't sleep for an entire night. On relating this story, she expressed emotion in the office for the first time. She did it easily, telling me "I never had anything like that before."

She has stopped worrying about her husband when he is away, has become calmer riding in the car with him at the wheel, and has become much less defensive with him and much more open, stating with finality "this wall is gone."

The dermatitis symptoms improved gradually, with small relapses along the way. For 2 1/2 years I gave no doses of any remedy. In the spring of 1989, two years after the Anthracinum, she experienced "no hay fever symptoms at all." Her premenstrual syndrome completely cleared up. However, she was diagnosed with cervical dysplasia and had a cone biopsy. Then her premenstrual syndrome came back, and the picture at that time fit Sepia. Really, the premenstrual syndrome was her only symptom. Strong irritability was the main characteristic, which felt much better from fast-paced walking. She also craved chocolate and, for four months, spotted in the two days before the onset of the menses.

She was given Sepia in May 1989. Afterwards, the premenstrual symptoms completely went away and her PAP smear became normal. Then, the eczema got worse and has been more of a problem over the last nine months. She's no longer my patient since I moved to Hawaii, but she is being followed by an able homeopath who keeps me abreast of the changes in her case. At this point, she may be moving toward Sulphur or Tuberculinum or perhaps needs more Anthracinum. But, in any case, she is remarkably improved in many ways since Anthracinum, and her symptomatology is focused on her skin and is not nearly as bothersome as before.

Case Number 3

Female, Age 40

March 24, 1988

She was bitten on her right tibia by a spider last summer, after which her entire calf and tibial area swelled up. Concurrently, her toes became quite cold. As a small child, she had strong reactions to spider bites. "They were like carbuncles."

Two weeks ago, she felt herself being bit but saw no bug. The pattern is that, first, there is a little dimple smaller than a flea bite; then it itches, swells (2), and hurts. The larger ones burn deep (3) inside and become "mean red" (3), toward purple; then a "crater" (ulcer) develops. She has numerous "bites" (3) on her legs (3), abdomen (2), and arms (1), but she's never seen an insect. The bites are mainly on her trunk, which is clothed. (The injuries section of Anthracinum in Hering's Guiding Symptoms says "after suspicious stings, if swelling changes color.")

No one else in her family has these bites. She lives with her family in the country, and they are surrounded by bugs. She has been living in the same valley for ten years. Until the bite on her anterior left ankle in 1986, she doesn't recall having this problem. This current bite is by far the worst it's ever been.

Medical History: A lump was removed from her right breast in November 1987. The lump developed after she was hit by a snow ball; she had a tingling sensation. It turned out to be a fibrocystic mass. She had eczema during lactation (3) with the first and second children. Her hands didn't even function; they cracked and bled (2).

Dairy foods cause flatulence and dry skin (1), not to the same extent as when she was lactating. It doesn't take a great deal of dairy to make her symptomatic.

Dry skin during menstrual cycle, after ovulation (1).

Slow metabolism; everything goes through slowly.

Constipates easily; has to "stay on top of it" to have a bowel movement once a day.

Desires salt (2), butter (3), and sweets (3).

"No interest sexually (3), none," for the last six months. After further questioning, she said it was not an aversion and admitted that her sex drive has been gone since the breast surgery (3).

She is hurried; "I speed (2) and I speed very naturally." Sugar really intensifies this hurriedness (2); leads to racing. "It (sugar) makes me uncomfortable, and 45 minutes later I'm one sad girl." Fruit juices are the worst (2).

Menses are normal; 31-day cycle; fairly regular. She is irritable before menses (2) for two days. "Easy to pick a fight and be irritable with the kids." After further questioning, she said that the irritability goes away about two days after onset of flow, that the menses itself is fine, and that the best time of month is mid-cycle.

The loss of her second child six years ago was a big grief. "I still haven't gotten over it...bitter (2)...still angry at them (medical system)...there went my perfect family." (Very upset and weeping.) Regrets (2) not having seen the baby.

Sleeps very well; starts on the right side (2); then ends up on her back to support her low back, which she injured in the past. Stays under the covers.

Loves the sun (2) and heat.

Needs gloves and hat to tolerate the cold (1).

She is a little photophobic (1); she squints in the sun (2) and wears sunglasses when driving.

She is anxious about her husband if he's late, and about her children in certain situations. She is also anxious about others (2), "sudden worst-case scenario." Comes up about once a week.

Thirstless (1).

Assessment: Allergic reaction to insect bites; grief.

Plan: Anthracinum 200c. Return to clinic in one month.

Analysis of Case Number 3

This time it was as if the fog and mist had completely cleared. I had no difficulty in perceiving the Anthracinum image and no qualms whatsoever in making the prescription. Not only was there a history of carbuncles from an early age (that was the word she used in describing them), but there was also a history of cracking dermatitis, which I had learned to associate with Anthracinum. Moreover, her presenting complaint was a bad reaction to insect bites, which Anthracinum is known for (it's italicized in the repertory). The premenstrual tension, particular food desires, anxiety regarding her husband, and history of grief were further indications and confirmations for Anthracinum.

Follow-Up on Case Number 3

First Follow-Up: May 17, 1988

Although she was to have returned for follow-up in one month, almost four months elapsed before I saw her.

"The remedy has done something. It's been different."

The third day after she took the remedy, she was "so sick, just down for the count...*felt so bad.*" Overall, she was not well; needing to sleep, and feeling tingly and nauseated, but not flu-like. Alternating between too hot and cold. "My whole self was sick; didn't want to ask for help. Just wanted to go down, to be sick, and it only lasted one day. By the next day, I was me, though not perfectly well." (So, once again, there's the organism retreating into a cocoon to heal.)

She's had only one bite that's scarred since then. Now, bites stay very, very localized and defined; don't spread out and get puffy.

Had a scratch in her ear, which she believes she made with her fingernail. While she was sick, the scratched area in her ear and the surrounding lymphatics swelled very much. The ear drained and wept for a whole month; white and green pus along with flakes. The sores on her legs became weepy. First they localized, walled off, and then drained green pus for an entire month every time she pressed.

She feels on the verge of crying and is more emotional in general. Before, "I had more control."

"I have more clarity, see more cause and effect in my life. I see that I have more choices."

The incision on her breast looks better. The last three days it's been burning. It has burned in the past, but this is the only time since the remedy.

There has been a minuscule improvement in her sexual drive. She believes that her sexual drive decreased after the incision in her breast (1).

She is in a workshop with a psychotherapist because of a dysfunctional family and her upbringing. Lost her nine-year-old sister when she was 13 years old, and also has "tremendous bitterness (3)" around the death of her child.

She has had two regular and good menstrual cycles; no problems at all with her skin; didn't notice any dry skin after ovulation.

She is very happy about her physical progress; she got a bite last weekend, which resolved on its own.

Assessment: "I'm very content!!" (again)

Plan: No remedy. Return to clinic in three months.

Second Follow-Up: August 16, 1988

She is very grateful; everything is working out fine.

Gets "bites here and there and they go. Now, they run the course of an ordinary bite."

The feelings of bitterness over her lost child "are settling." She believes these feelings tie into herself as a child and all she's experienced in her life, especially her sister's death, "a bitter, sad event," and the breakup of her family.

Her sexual drive has increased, "but it's slow."

She is more satisfied with her life in general.

Has come to realize that her speeding isn't healthy; doesn't want it and now is able to say "no," do a little less, and be more content.

"It feels like I've lost pieces which weren't important — chunks of me which I don't miss."

Assessment: The Anthracinum has produced a wonderfully deep effect.

Plan: No remedy. Discharged; return to the clinic as needed.

Case Number 4

I have another case where Anthracinum produced a significant effect. I had been treating this woman for three years. First, I gave her Aurum metallicum (with beautiful results) for depression with suicidal tendencies. Then, she developed dermatitis on her hands, similar to the other cases. It first manifested with a rash on her right palm, on the forefinger of her left hand, and on her left foot. It was very itchy, and was made worse from scratching and rubbing. This was a bad dermatitis, much worse than in Case Number 2. It was mostly on her fingers. She was attending college and couldn't even write. She had used a topical salve with no results.

Her depression was now minor compared to what it had been. I was reluctant to treat her, but she insisted. I gave her a dose of Sulphur 30c, but the effect wasn't lasting. She had cravings for sweets, thirst for cold drinks, uncovering and covering in bed, and fear of heights. After the Sulphur, her dermatitis got much better but then got worse again and began to spread. She got bubbles, fluid-filled and watery. I wouldn't treat her for a while after that. I just talked with her at length about the principles of cure and told her what I thought was going on.

Many months later, I gave her a dose of Rhus toxicodendron 30c. It helped her a little, but then she gradually got worse again. Several months later she demanded, "You have to treat me or I will take cortisone. This thing is driving me crazy. I just want to give it a last shot. I want a high potency; no fooling around." I looked at her. She is very heavy and yet refined. The lesions were really dry and cracking. I asked her if she had any sebaceous cysts. She showed me one on her right thigh; it was hard and large.

I gave her Anthracinum 200c. A letter arrived two months later:

...The results of the remedy have been so dramatic that I am still reeling. I took the medication 7 a.m., Thursday, April 9th. During that afternoon it seemed to me my hand was improved.... On Friday evening the open cracks were healed over. I could open and close my hand without discomfort.

On Saturday, a dull headache on waking. In the afternoon, a close look at my hand showed that the fluid sacks beneath the skin were disappearing.... In reverse order, the eruptions on my feet were resolving...a definite sense of calm, *bliss*. There is no heat, no cracking, no opening of the skin, no swelling, no bleeding; just the presence of dead skin. There is only one small amount of activity.... The skin on the hand got much better, but then it got worse again and things began to spread. There remain two small areas. Today there was a tiny spot on the hand. There is such a feeling of bliss. I hope that the other two spots give up and go the way of the rest of their brothers.

As an aside, I have perceived no mental/emotional alterations at this time, but I am in a state of intense serenity. I have been so tickled about the physical symptoms that this may have blocked my awareness of the mental/emotional symptoms, but seriously I do not believe that there were any mental/emotional symptoms.

I am unable to provide you with extended follow-up in this case because she moved far away to take a teaching position. But clearly this is another example of Anthracinum acting with a good effect.

The Common Thread: A Pathogenesis of Anthracinum

I'd like to share with you my pathogenesis for Anthracinum in order to help you understand how such a remedy image evolves and to shed more light on the relationship between Anthracinum's physical and psychological characteristics.

Remember, the patients described here are basically happy people; they said so themselves. Yet, something is awry inside. They probably won't spontaneously complain or volunteer any information on their emotional states unless they are asked. And then you may get a story about a big grief, from which they have effectively disconnected themselves. It's as if their emotional fabric has an invisible wall in itself. In a way, this wall serves them well in that they are happy, but it fails to put them in touch with dormant emotional issues that are clearly unresolved.

It's as if on some unconscious level each person has made the decision to be selfless, rather than to confront their wounded self and attempt to heal it. In all three cases they have been forsaken at some point in their lives. In Case Number 1, the husband left; in Case Number 2, the father died; and in Case Number 3, the sister died and, later, she lost a child. But, curiously, she didn't even think to mention the loss of her sister until after Anthracinum had been given. So, again, the idea of disconnecting from a painful experience is present.

In all three instances, huge losses occurred early in life, and then an interesting set of psycho- and physiodynamic phenomena took place. You could say that the ego or the self got walled off, much like a tuberculous granuloma gets walled off to protect the organism. Under these circumstances, the personality at the time could not cope with the stress. So, it ceased to expand, and a compensatory self-protective mechanism intervened on behalf of the vital force.

The women in the first two cases did not harden around their griefs, as you might expect to see in Natrum muriaticum, Ignatia, Aurum, or Causticum. Instead, you could say they gave in to it or softened around it. After taking Anthracinum, the "soft tissue" surrounding the grief broke down, much like Silicea promotes actual physical suppuration. But, in these cases, the discharge took place on the emotional level, allowing for a great release and elimination of the now unwanted foreign body — *the grief itself*, which previously had never been processed.

The grief then becomes identified, processed, accepted for what it represents, and finally expelled. I believe this event allows for the resumption of healthier psychological development, wherein future experiences, especially on the emotional level, may be directly and freely integrated. What parallels this so beautifully is the physical analog — the cyst, the tumor, or the carbuncle that opens and relieves itself under the influence of Anthracinum.

I'd like to make several other points. These patients are very family-oriented people. The anxiety they experience concerning their husbands relates to the unresolved grief and abandonment in their pasts. The husband represents a pillar of support, so the mere thought that his safety is threatened in any way poses a threat to their entire world. Having known the families of all three women, I can also say that these patients are strongly bothered by disharmony in their environment, especially the noise of shouting.

They are fast-moving people, not impatient, but quick to grasp (Ignatia). They seem to be quite refined, with rather delicate features (Silicea). They may be sweet, unassertive, very sensitive, and proper. They may not have a very strong sense of themselves. They lack self-confidence, can be hard on themselves (self-reproach), and need to be in control.

Although they may not complain about sexual function, they have all improved markedly in this area after Anthracinum. So, there must be a relationship between sexual dysfunction and the imprinting of grief.

Don't forget the following symptoms and characteristics that Anthracinum addressed in at least two of the cases I've presented:

- Fear of being alone (two of three).
- Anxiety about others, especially husband (all three).
- Allergies: hay fever, petroleum products, insect bites (all three).
- Premenstrual syndrome with irritability (two of three).
- Love of the sun; skin problems may be ameliorated by the sun (all three).
- Photophobia (two of three).
- Craving for sweets (all three).

Finally, the remedies you are most likely to confuse with Anthracinum are Silicea, Natrum muriaticum, Pulsatilla, and Aurum. Look for the characteristic types of Anthracinum symptoms on the physical level to help you, especially cysts, carbuncles, and dry, cracking dermatitis. I've given the remedy in three other cases where the mental and emotional states fit but none of the physical symptoms that seem to characterize the remedy were present. In each case, Anthracinum had no effect. So, I think it's safe to say that Anthracinum is not a substitute for Natrum muriaticum when the patient has a need to be in control, a history of grief, is chilly, and craves sweets rather than salt. Some of the other characteristic Anthracinum indications must also be present.

Baker: Would anyone like to share an Anthracinum case from your practice?

Stephen King: Since I first heard you present a preliminary version of this information several years ago, I have used Anthracinum successfully in two cases. One case in particular is noteworthy. The patient was a young man in his early 30s — tall, thin, Silicea-like in appearance. He was somewhat shy, artistic, refined, and articulate.

He came to see me for help with a severe case of cystic acne and dermatitis. His entire back looked like a battle zone. It was covered with large, angry pustules, involving deeper skin layers, and with scars, craters, birthmarks, and moles. There were also a number of lesions on the buttocks and thighs. This skin problem had begun around puberty. The man had suffered with it for about 20 years, despite numerous courses of antibiotics and other conventional treatments.

Much of his younger life had been spent in Southeast Asia, where his father worked as an engineer. He had many immunizations, which may have been a factor in his condition.

On an emotional plane, my patient had never felt very supported by his family. He felt that he was on the outside looking in, forsaken by his family. Consequently, as an adult, he was desperately looking for a love relationship that would give meaning to his life. Being independent was difficult, despite much psychotherapy.

He also had a history of orchitis. I first prescribed Aurum metallicum, which had no effect. I thought about Natrum muriaticum but was troubled by the fact that he loved the sun. Then I remembered your earlier presentation, in which you described Anthracinum's similarity to Natrum muriaticum, but with Anthracinum being chillier and liking the sun.

I prescribed Anthracinum 200c about three years ago. A gradual yet remarkable improvement has taken place. The patient says his skin is approximately 90 percent better. He still has a few lesions. The skin has also become softer, more flexible, and less indurated so that the remaining lesions are more superficial. The remedy has been repeated about three times.

Anthracinum has also produced some very positive emotional changes. He has become more independent and more able to stand on his own. He is no longer driven by a desperate need to be in a relationship.

Baker: *That's a wonderful case. Thanks very much.*

Conclusion

Beyond the information I've presented, I think there are a few good lessons here. First, take very thorough cases. If a well-known remedy doesn't emerge, keep digging. You might find precious metal in a previously untapped mine. Second, allow the remedies you give to act—*fully.* Don't change remedies until all the curative potential, all the good of that substance, has exhausted itself. Third, be equally thorough on follow-up. Even if you've prescribed on what appears to be only a superficial basis, be aware of deeper symptoms and changes that may tip you off to new aspects and hitherto unknown facets of that remedy.

Remember, if we're not looking we'll never see. Dare to be great. Consider this: If, just once or twice in our careers, each one of us perceives fresh new information that sheds clear light on the character of remedies previously unrevealed, the cumulative effect will be stupendous. Potentially, immense amounts of valuable new material will be generated. This material will enable homeopaths everywhere to be more effective and ultimately will make homeopathy an even more powerful medicine than it is today.

Michael Carlston, MD, DHt

A CASE OF UNSTABLE ANGINA PECTORIS

Michael Carlston, MD, DHt, was first introduced to homeopathy by Dr. Rudolph Ballentine. His teachers have included George Vithoulkas, Maesie Panos, Bill Gray, Roger Morrison, and Vassilis Ghegas. He is a graduate of the University of Minnesota Medical School and completed his Family Practice residency in 1984 at Bethesda Lutheran Medical Center. From 1982 to 1985, Michael was a clinical instructor in the Department of Family Practice and Community Health at the University of Minnesota. He completed the IFH Professional Course in 1985 and received his DHt in 1988. He first practiced homeopathy in Minneapolis and then moved to Santa Rosa, where he now practices at the Annadel Clinic of Natural Medicine.

Some Introductory Remarks on the Role of the Homeopath

My purpose in presenting this case is to ease our anxiety about patients with organic heart disease. You *can* help these people. As John Clarke wrote in his *Diseases of the Heart and Arteries:*

In the vocabulary of medicine there is no term more charged with fatal import to the lay mind than that of heart disease. It means, in the language of the laity, a disease that is incurable, and that is sure to end in sudden death sooner or later. Now this is very far from being the truth. Heart disease is not by any means incurable; many forms of it are capable of being perfectly cured; and in others a practical cure may be effected through compensatory increase of strength, even when the damaged part does not itself admit of repair.

I hope to make a broader point as well. We homeopaths have isolated ourselves from other physicians for too long. While isolation may once have been the best strategy for survival, times have changed. People are becoming increasingly open to considering different ways to live their lives. They are also becoming more aware of the long-term effects of their actions in the world — an ecological sensitivity in a way. We see these changes every day around us. This shift brings the mainstream of our society closer to a homeopathic world view. Homeopathy is growing more rapidly now than ever before in the United States. Although we physicians tend to be more resistant to change than are our patients, there is a marked increase in physician interest in homeopathy. In this climate of exploration, isolation hurts homeopathy.

I am among the first to agree that the greatest good is achieved by preventing serious illness. Homeopathy is uniquely gifted in its ability to strengthen the individual, thereby helping people become healthier than ever before. On the other hand, people occasionally have a need for hospitalization, despite the very best homeopathic care. Almost all of us will certainly find ourselves one day with patients in the hospital. Allopathic medicine has made great strides in emergency-hospital medical care over the years, but homeopathy still has something to add.

American homeopaths in the last century were "real" doctors. They were primary care physicians, not specialist consultants as we tend to be today. Their patients turned to them for aid, no matter what the diagnosis, so homeopaths had the opportunity to treat a wide variety of pathology. They reported routine cures of diseases that would terrify most of us because we lack their experience and, perhaps, because we might not believe homeopathy can cure such "serious illnesses."

The time has come to reclaim our heritage. It has been so wonderful to witness the changes since my introduction to homeopathy 17 years ago. We should celebrate the tremendous advances of recent years. Then, we should chart a course toward higher goals. I believe that, if we set our wills to it, we will be able to start homeopathic wings in hospitals across the country in the next 15 years. When the day arrives that you wake to find yourself unexpectedly in the hospital, wouldn't it be nice to look up and see familiar faces? How about opening hospitals that have been designed as true healing environments and, better still, homeopathic in approach?

We have a great opportunity now to lift homeopathy to its rightful station in American health care. To achieve this goal, each of us must decide what more she or he can do. Try to become more visible in your community. Reach out to allopathic doctors. Apply for hospital privileges.

Some allopaths believe that we have horns and tails. They are mistaken. Equally mistaken are homeopaths who think allopaths are evil because they aren't homeopaths. Homeopaths who believe that most allopaths would never refer patients to them are also mistaken. We homeopaths must not be the faction maintaining the barrier that keeps us apart. If the Berlin Wall can come down so easily, then why not the wall between us and allopathic medicine? If American physicians are truly dedicated to healing, there is no reason whatsoever for this barrier to exist.

Background on the Patient

I.H.K.
Female
Born: June 10, 1912

This is the case of a 77-year-old woman who became my patient in September 1988. At that time, she had a number of relatively minor health complaints, in addition to suffering from severely arthritic knees. She was due to have a second knee replacement in two weeks and hoped that I might be able to aid her healing from the surgery. She was dedicated to homeopathy ever since she had been helped by a homeopath decades ago for a severe allergy problem. Like many others, she believed that homeopathy was effective but completely harmless and thus used remedies quite freely for any troubles she experienced.

My impression of her was that she paid an undue amount of attention to minor health difficulties. Other than arthritis, digestive troubles were her most prevalent problem, particularly bloating and continual hunger. As a child, while living in Tanganyika, she had malaria and tsetse fever. In the 1930s she was diagnosed hypothyroid, for which she took medication (later I discovered that her thyroid pills were "homeopathic" thyroid pills). The tests I ordered of her thyroid function were always normal. She discontinued her thyroid pills at my direction in March 1989. It is of note that her father and siblings died of heart disease.

The first time I saw Ms. K. I found that her heart rate was quite slow (52), although regular. This was usual for her, she said. In addition, I found a III/VI systolic ejection murmur at her left sternal border. The EKG at that time revealed only sinus bradycardia. Other times her EKG showed atrial fibrillation, once with rapid ventricular response. She is a very pleasant elderly woman with a classic Lycopodium body type: heavy through the hips, disproportionate to her upper body size.

The knee surgery went well, but she required general anesthesia several months later to allow manipulation to release the adhesions that developed in her knee. Prior to the surgery, I had given her Arsenicum album 12c daily as a chronic prescription, without effect. Following surgery, I prescribed Arnica for her knee pain, and then Lycopodium for the knee pain and her chronic troubles. Both acted well, and the Lycopodium helped her chronic complaints. When Lycopodium stopped helping her, I prescribed Magnesia carbonica, which somewhat relieved her. Finally, I prescribed Silicea just before her crisis occurred.

An Emergency Hospitalization for Angina

August 11, 1989

The patient's cholesterol was 243.

August 13, 1989

The patient experienced severe substernal chest pain at 7:30 a.m., with associated severe diaphoresis (profuse perspiration), nausea, and palpitations. After two hours of intense symptoms, the nausea, diaphoresis, and palpitations ceased, and the chest pain became less severe. She left a message with the answering service for me to call her the next day (Monday). They realized that it shouldn't wait, so they called me.

She didn't feel that hospitalization was necessary, but she agreed to try some nitroglycerin. The first dose did nothing. The second dose partially alleviated her pain. Then I convinced her of the necessity for hospitalization. At the time that I admitted her to the Intensive Care Unit (ICU) of Community Hospital in Santa Rosa she continued to experience a low level of the same pressure-like chest pain. She recalled two similar episodes of pain. The first was one month earlier while walking up a steep hill on Alcatraz Island, and the other occurred in the week before admission, also while walking.

Physical Examination: She was remarkably calm, considering the circumstances and the ICU environment.

- Mild hypotension (100-122/60-88).
- Sinus bradycardia (48-54). Sometimes sinus irregularity was present.
- III-IV/VI systolic ejection murmur at the left sternal border.
- No signs of failure.
- EKG: Sinus bradycardia. Otherwise, no significant changes.
- Lab: Hemoglobin 10.7. Sodium 134. Alkaline phosphatase elevated. Otherwise, normal including cardiac enzymes.
- Chest x-ray: Normal for her age (calcified aorta).

Obtained a cardiologist consultation.

Hospital Course

The patient was treated with the usual Coronary Care Unit protocols, including heparinization, but not prophylactic lidocaine. Her pain was helped with nitrates, but she often required morphine as well. She also noticed that her pain was helped by warm drinks.

August 17, 1989

Ms. K.'s heart was catheterized because, as the cardiologist feared, even the newest available calcium channel blocker (Cardene) did not adequately control her pain. The catheterization revealed hypercritical right main coronary artery disease (99 percent occluded) and moderate proximal left coronary occlusion (70 percent). The right main coronary artery was a very small vessel, only about 2 mm in diameter.

August 19, 1989

A stress test was performed. The patient was unable to exercise to capacity because of fatigue and discomfort in the extremities, only achieving two miles per hour on a 12 percent grade. She had no chest pain during the test. Thus, the test was inadequate.

Lab: Ms. K.'s low hemoglobin was evaluated without significant findings. Her alkaline phosphatase was elevated, certainly because of her arthritis and resultant knee replacements.

Plan: Although her pain was still not entirely under control, the cardiologists felt that nothing further could be done for her in the hospital, so she was discharged on Isordil 20 mg by mouth three times per day, Cardene 20 mg by mouth three times per day, and nitroglycerin 1/150 sublingual as needed for chest pain. The dietician recommended continuation of her low-salt, low-cholesterol diet. I asked her to see me in one week.

Symptoms Are Poorly Controlled with Conventional Medications

August 25, 1989

Still using many nitroglycerin: five yesterday.

Cardene 20 mg three times per day and Isordil 20 mg three times per day.

Chest pain (1); maximum intensity 3/10. Weight in the center of her chest (1); does not radiate.

A headache occurs with the pain (1). Left-sided (2). Uncertain if the headache occurs only after taking the nitroglycerin.

Palpitations (1), sometimes occur with the headache and chest pain.

Legs feel heavy (1), "...like lead in my veins (2)."

Constipated (2).

Desires warm drinks (3).

Dry mouth (1).

The cardiologist wanted to try an experimental drug that has only a number and not yet a name. "Isn't there something homeopathic you can try?" asked Ms. K.

Physical Examination:
- Weight: 148 lbs.
- Cardiovascular: Regular, with systolic ejection murmur as before.

Assessment: Continued unstable angina.

At this point I was frustrated and concerned. I felt helpless. I had failed because one of my patients had started on allopathic drugs while under my care, and now the cardiologist wanted to put her on an experimental drug. Add to this stew the pleas of a very sweet elderly woman for help. I decided that, hoping against hope, I might as well give it a try for the honor of homeopathy. Why not? I asked her to wait two more weeks. I think the reason I had her wait was to be certain that two more weeks on the Cardene and Isordil wouldn't take care of her angina. Of course, that would also allow me time to build up my courage to give her the remedy she appeared to need.

Plan: Return in two weeks.

September 8, 1989

Using one to seven nitroglycerin a day. Average is six per day. So far this morning she
   has used four.

Chest pains occur at any time (2).

Left-sided (2) headache, might be before she takes the nitroglycerin.

Constipated (2).

Pain in the right mid-upper arm (1) at the base of the deltoid.

Incontinent of urine; worse under stress (cough or sneeze) (3). Old symptom since a
   urinary tract infection in February 1988.

Very affected by colors and music (1).

Wants to be alone (1).

Noticing a pulsing in her neck; the right side is better than the left.

Chilly (2).

Desires sweets, salt, cheese, and bitter (2).

Physical examination:
   • Weight: 143 1/4 lbs.
   • Blood Pressure: 118/56 (right arm).

Assessment: Unstable angina.

By this time it was clear that something had to be done. She was continuing to
experience angina, despite maximum medical therapy, and appeared to be facing an
inevitable myocardial infarction. Although the area of heart muscle she would lose
would be rather limited, the tissue involved seemed to be important electrically
because of the palpitations she experienced with her angina. Dilatation of a vessel this
size (2 mm) would be difficult, so angioplasty wouldn't be a good option either. What
could we do? Which remedy would you choose?

Durr Elmore: It seems as if you didn't have much to diagnose from, and you probably wanted a heart remedy. I thought of Spigelia. It has left-sided symptoms. It has left-sided headaches and the desire for warm, or hot, drinks.

Steve Olsen: One remedy to consider for angina and heart disease is Haematoxylon, or logwood. It covers many of the symptoms that one would expect with this type of condition: sense of constriction, sensation of a bar laying across the chest, and angina pectoris. Something to consider.

Audience: One other point for Spigelia is the small rubric, "nausea during the pain." There are only a few remedies for this rubric, and Spigelia is on page 509 under, "STOMACH, nausea during pain."

Andrea Sullivan: I thought of Cactus for the angina pectoris. As a student, I had a patient who had angina on exertion. She was a very pleasant, elderly African-American woman — not at all like the mental and emotional picture for angina.

Carlston: Anybody else? Any other remedies to consider?

Audience: Naja, because it's an important angina remedy.

Peggy Chipkin: This is a real wild shot, but I was impressed with the calmness of the patient in the emergency room. Also, she had recent surgery. I just looked up Arnica. "Says there's nothing wrong with him," which is how she was acting there. Boericke strongly alludes to Arnica for angina.

Homeopathic Analysis of the Case

I considered several remedies, namely Phosphorus, Argentum nitricum, Lachesis, Bryonia, and Cactus. Phosphorus was considered for very little reason except that she had palpitations and a very friendly, warm personality. Her amelioration from warm drinks, however, practically eliminated Phosphorus from serious consideration. Argentum nitricum was considered on the strength of her palpitations with the chest pain, but it just didn't suit her the way a good prescription should.

Lachesis was often in my mind because of the totality of heart symptoms, the gastrointestinal trouble, and the peculiar complaint of "heaviness, like lead in my veins." Her tendency toward loquacity, the left-sided headache, desire to be alone, and sensitivity to colors and music intensified my interest in Lachesis. Earlier in the case she had a peculiar symptom that Lachesis is known to have. This symptom is a very tight anus, requiring her to pull her buttocks apart to pass gas. However, I hesitated to use Lachesis because of her strong desire for and amelioration by warm drinks, and because of the disparity between the Lachesis mental state that I would expect in such a severe case and the pleasant, emotionally balanced person in front of me.

I liked the idea of Bryonia. It suited her overall, matching many of her specific complaints. It can be helpful in heart conditions. On the other hand, its action isn't so intensely focused on cardiac function, and, more importantly, I could not elicit any of the typical Bryonia modalities from her. For example, if the palpitations were brought on by motion or the headache were ameliorated by pressure, I would have considered Bryonia as a stronger possibility.

Cactus was a good thought because this patient's pathology was almost entirely focused on her heart, and Cactus is one of our most profoundly effective remedies for heart conditions. It is known also for headaches, although they tend to be right-sided. Her heart symptoms suited Cactus fairly well: weight in the center of the chest and palpitations. I could not, despite my attempts to do so, confirm that her pains were the usual constrictive Cactus-type of cardiac pain, nor were her palpitations of the usual sort for Cactus, radiating to the left arm and aggravated by lying on the left side.

The lack of specific modalities and the overall lack of information led me to realize that this case would be either quite simple or practically impossible. I expected the latter.

The Remedy Is Found and Prescribed

As she was relating her complaints to me, I felt frustrated by the lack of solid, reliable symptoms. I decided to throw out everything in the case except what I knew. Then I could explore the possible remedies from a firm base of symptomatology. I was then left with constipation, pain in the upper right arm, a strong desire for warm drinks, stress-related incontinence, palpitations, and a weight-like chest pain. The best symptom was the one she had given me in the hospital, that her chest pain was better from warm drinks. Unfortunately, that symptom isn't in Kent's repertory. In addition, she had headaches that probably were independent of the nitroglycerin, but they were definitely left-sided.

How about Spigelia anthelmia? Demerara pinkroot (not Carolina pinkroot, which is Spigelia marylandia) grows throughout Central and South America. It received its European name in honor of a countess who was famed for using it and other substances to poison people. It was introduced into European pharmacological use as a vermifuge in 1751 by a physician named Patrick Browne. Hahnemann, who proved it along with 13 other remedies in 1819, discovered its powerful cardiac effects.

I knew that Spigelia has left-sided headaches in addition to its cardiac effects, but I didn't know the remedy well. So, I quickly reviewed some of my books. In Boericke's description of heart symptoms I found "violent palpitation," "angina pectoris," and, in one of those all too rare moments when you are seeking a strange symptom, "craving for hot water which relieves." Except for Phatak, who acknowledges Boericke as a source, I have been unable to find this symptom in any of the published material on Spigelia. Pierre Schmidt added "desire for warm drinks with angina" to Kent's repertory. The patient was unable to confirm any other Spigelia symptoms, but I felt hopeful because of this most peculiar characteristic of her angina.

Plan: I gave her one dose of Spigelia 30c in my office. As the patient observed herself over the passage of time, it became clear that she experienced many of the classic features of Spigelia. As we all know, hindsight is "20/20."

September 12, 1989

The cardiologist was feeling frustrated with her lack of improvement. He sent me a letter describing his evaluation of the patient. His closing line was, "I certainly hope that we'll be able to find a good medical regimen for her." This did not encourage me to believe that he would. It is interesting that he attributed her headaches to nitroglycerin, a natural assumption, I suppose. Also, he seemed to have found little reassurance in the fact that, since taking the Spigelia three days before, she had been free of angina!

September 21, 1989

The patient called me and reported the following:

After taking the remedy, she didn't need any nitroglycerin for three days (3).

Stopped Procardia (new prescription) because she didn't like the way she felt while taking it.

The cardiologist had stopped the Cardene.

Had already stopped Isordil on her own.

Overall is definitely better (1).

Horrible constipation (3).

Plan: She said she was feeling much better. I was delighted. The reason for her call was to report her difficulty with constipation, but I had enough wisdom to know that it is better to have constipation than heart disease. So, I told her to wait.

The Patient Relapses

September 25, 1989

She called because her angina had returned quite severely. It was only 17 days after the initial dose.

Plan: I instructed her to take one dose of Spigelia 200c.

September 27, 1989

Cardiologist: "The history of angina and particularly its frequency is more than a little bit discouraging... I'll keep my fingers crossed."

The patient had her relapse just prior to her appointment with the cardiologist. She was wrestling with an ethical issue now. Should she risk alienating her cardiologist by telling him that she wasn't taking his medicine and, worse still, feeling better? Later on, she told him everything in more detail than he was willing to hear.

Further Improvement and Then She Panics

October 2, 1989

She had taken 10 nitroglycerin on September 24. Since she took the remedy on September 25 she has used only six nitroglycerin (0,3,1,1,1,0,0). None yet today.

Heart pounds (1); ameliorated when lying on her back or right side (1).

Constipation.

Dizzy; worse in the morning.

Gums hurt. Metallic taste in her mouth.

Pain in the right arm (1).

Desires salt (2).

Unrefreshed sleep.

Dislikes the constriction of her bra.

Physical Examination: Chest clear; pulse regular.

Assessment: The patient's report at this visit was quite impressive. Again, the Spigelia had clearly and dramatically acted to alleviate her angina. I was delighted, but I was also watching vigilantly for another remedy to appear. My experience with small remedies has indicated that, after a period of time (generally less than six months), the patient frequently moves on to a more common remedy pattern. The clear consideration here was Lachesis because of the palpitations that were ameliorated by lying on the right side, the aversion to constrictive clothing, and the unrefreshed sleep.

The wise homeopath knows when to think about great ideas for the next remedy but only to contemplate and not to act. Clearly, the best course was to allow her to continue on this path of progressive improvement. Spigelia is known for difficulty in breathing, ameliorated by lying on the right side. This symptom is attributed to hydrothorax in the reported cases. One or two authors also imply an amelioration of palpitations by resting on the right side, but I could find no clear declaration to confirm this.

October 5, 1989

Homeopaths often become impatient and spoil a case by over treatment. Ms. K. panicked and gave herself another dose of Spigelia 200c. She experienced the temporary malaise that commonly follows in such circumstances.

The Patient Continues To Do Well on Spigelia

November 3, 1989

Since October 4, she has had 20 days without requiring any nitroglycerin. She has taken 13 nitroglycerin in 30 days (3): six days with one only, three days demanding two, and one day needing three.

"Overall feeling much better (2)."

Dizziness in her head and legs. Objects seem to move from right to left; legs are a bit wobbly. Worse in the morning (1).

Pain in the right upper arm; sometimes in the left. Worse when at rest.

Legs feel tired.

Generally ameliorated with warm drinks (2) (long, prevalent pattern).

Constipation is much better (2).

Lip margins are rough.

Desires salt (2).

Assessment: By the visit on November 3 it was clear that Spigelia was more than a homeopathic Glonoine or nitroglycerin for her. It was not just an acute remedy. It was acting to help her heal a broad range of her symptoms. She told me at this visit that warm drinks ameliorated her generally, not only the anginal symptoms. Lachesis slid further from my mind, to be replaced by Chelidonium and Bryonia. Her nitroglycerin usage had dropped now to a consistently low level, averaging one every other day from her pre-Spigelia level of six per day.

I observed with this patient what Clarke also observed, "I have again and again noticed this effect of Spigelia in relieving constipation in cardiac patients to whom I have been giving it." Each of the Spigelia cases he described in his *Diseases of the Heart and Arteries* experienced dizziness as did Ms. K., and most of his cases had anxiety, as did my patient. He found Spigelia to be the most useful remedy in cases of alcohol- or nicotine-induced heart disease.

The Angina Returns

December 7, 1989

On December 2, the patient called complaining of chest pain with dizziness, including a sensation of "dizziness in the chest." Nitroglycerin did not ease her pain. She then took Spigelia 200c at my direction. Shortly thereafter, her symptoms abated. In the past two weeks, her angina was becoming more frequent again.

New chest pains; on December 1, stitching pain in the heart transiently.

Sometimes constrictive sensation under her breasts. Occurs while sitting and lying, especially when lying on the left side. Loosening her bra doesn't help.

Pain in the right shoulder; worse at night.

Her heels hurt because of shoes.

Unsteady; worse when walking slow (2) or fast.

Legs feel like lead, but not painful.

Fingernails are cracked and split.

Generally ameliorated with warm drinks (2). They help her to belch and lessen bloating, but belching doesn't ameliorate the chest pain.

Stool every other day.

Hands are always cold (1).

Physical Examination:
- Blood Pressure: 130/70.
- Cardiovascular System: Slightly bradycardic, but regular. No change in the murmur. Chest clear.

Plan: Obtain a serum cholesterol count.

Assessment: Six weeks after the Spigelia 200c, she needed another dose. It is interesting that the day before we repeated the dose she experienced the sharp heart pain that is classically associated with Spigelia. Upon questioning, she recalled that her pain at the time of her hospitalization, when it was at its most intense, was sharp at times, "like a stiletto." This knife-like pain is the most characteristic type of heart pain related to Spigelia. In his discussion of a case of pericarditis cured by Spigelia, Clarke writes, "The knife-like pain singled out Spigelia from all the other medicines related to this condition."

Plan: I felt at this point that she was doing passably well, but I was concerned that things seemed a bit shaky. So, I instructed her to have both Spigelia 200c and 1M on hand.

A Nitroglycerin Overdose and Another Hospitalization

December 19, 1989

The patient called. She had chest pain with the usual associated symptoms and took four nitroglycerin in one-half hour. After taking the nitroglycerin, her chest pain was better, but she was so light-headed that she fell to the floor, reinjuring her knee (most recent prosthesis). She then called me in severe pain from her knee. I instructed her to repeat the Spigelia 200c and to call her orthopedist regarding the possible damage to her prosthesis.

He hospitalized her for nursing support, pain control, and evaluation of her syncopal episode, and he consulted her cardiologist. I was unable to participate in her hospital care because the orthopedist put her in a hospital that I am not affiliated with. During the hospitalization she had a Thallium scan, which revealed nothing of significance. She also had a normal upper gastrointestinal series. The cardiologist agreed with me that the cause for her fall was the nitroglycerin overdose. He also felt that this proved that the homeopathic remedy did not work.

December 28, 1989

The cardiologist discharged the patient on Tenormin for her angina, aspirin for its antiplatelet activity, and Tylenol for the pain.

January 3, 1990

Feeling worse (2).

Dizziness much worse (2).

No nitroglycerin since hospitalization but she would "rather have heart pain than feel like this (1)."

Feels slow (3).

Pulse slow (3).

Chest pain; may be aggravated at rest.

Headache (1).

Pain in the right shoulder; worse at night.

Desires potatoes (3), salty (3), spicy (2).

Urinary incontinence (2).

Desires open air (1).

Physical Examination: Pulse 44 and regular.

Assessment: Her fall on December 19 was unfortunate. Her unacknowledged anxiety motivated her to take four doses of nitroglycerin over much too short a time, resulting in a syncopal spell and injury to her prosthesis.

In retrospect, it is clear that another Spigelia pattern ran through her case. That is, almost every severe episode of chest pain that she experienced occurred a short time after she got up in the morning. Dr. Gross observed in the original proving, "In the morning after rising from bed as soon as he sits down the heart begins to beat strongly, and above the place where it is felt beating a heavy, painfully pressing weight seems to lie which causes oppression..."

The Thallium scan found nothing, and she did not experience chest pain during the scan. Therefore, she had not infarcted any of her myocardium. Because none of his therapy had helped, the cardiologist felt she should try a beta-blocker (Tenormin), even though she tended to have bradycardia and low blood pressure. As a result, she felt quite poorly and the case was obscured.

Plan: Clearly, the beta-blocker should be discontinued. Although Tenormin has a long half-life and she had taken it for only a few days, I cautiously weaned her from it by cutting her dose to one-half for one week, then to one-third for another week before stopping it.

A Higher Potency of Spigelia is Required

January 7, 1990

The patient called because of a severe episode of chest pain, palpitation, extreme vertigo, and nausea, lasting for over two hours. She was unable to feel her pulse during the episode (2). One dose of nitroglycerin had not helped.

Plan: I instructed her to take one dose of Spigelia 1M and call me in one hour. She was much better within the hour, and by the evening was only moderately fatigued.

January 25, 1990

Decreased Tenormin as directed. None for 13 days. No nitroglycerin (2).

Lead feeling in legs "as if in the veins" is gone (2). Occasionally feels as if a slight weight is in her legs.

Fingers warmer and less numb than before the last dose of the remedy (1).

Bowels much better (2).

Dizziness much better (2), especially after a stool.

Headache much better (2). Sometimes occurs with constipation, other times immediately after stool.

Skin on legs not scaling as much (1).

No change in right upper arm pain (2), which is worse at night and while resting (1).

Worse in the morning (1).

Physical Examination:
- Weight: 145 lbs.
- Pulse: 54 and regular.
- Hands cold to touch.

Assessment: The patient was much improved (3). The episode on January 7 was quite frightening to both the patient and me. The degree of circulatory collapse she experienced with these episodes was extreme. Waiting for even one hour was difficult. Fortunately, she responded quickly.

On her January 25 visit I was delighted that she hadn't needed any nitroglycerin for 13 days. The peculiar symptom of a feeling of lead in her veins seemed to be temporally associated with times of increased angina. Although Spigelia is known for great weightiness and tearing pains in the legs, I have not found a written description of a similar sensation. I would be curious to know if anyone else has seen it. The peculiar symptom of vertigo, made better with a stool, is listed in Kent for Alumina, Cuprum, Lachesis, and Oenanthe. I once again resisted the idea of Lachesis.

Plan: Wait.

February 15, 1990

Chest pain was better. Only five nitroglycerin in the last three weeks. Pain with hurry.

Constrictive sensation at times.

Saw orthopedist on February 6. He diagnosed a cyst in her right shoulder and injected it with cortisone and Xylocaine. Less pain.

Still has some periods of weariness, but better.

Naps are helping.

Lead feeling in legs is gone (2). Some heaviness felt in knees only.

Fingers are still cool but better.

Little dizziness. Still unsteady.

Jittery with hunger (1).

Desires salt (2).

Occasional gum pain.

Nails brittle.

Almost no protein in her diet.

Physical Examination:
- Weight: 147 1/2 lbs.
- Blood Pressure: 122/76.
- Pulse: 60 and regular.

Assessment: Her unsteadiness and the fact that she was less disturbed by fast walking were probably due to loss of proprioception after her knee replacements. Interestingly, the cortisone injection didn't disturb the case. She differentiated between her heart pain and the constrictive sensation she felt in her lower chest. I felt that the case was changing and that she might need a different remedy soon.

Plan: Add more protein to the diet. Return in one month.

A New Remedy Is Given

March 19, 1990

Still uses about one nitroglycerin each week. Alleviates pain in less than one-half hour. No other medication since January 12.

Constipation is better (2).

Stool appears normal. Occasional incomplete stool. Must eat a lot of fruit to have a daily bowel movement.

Two headaches a week. One type is a frontal headache from constipation (2), more than once a week, and has other headaches sometimes, which are occipital, not left-sided.

Chest pain only when carrying heavy objects (3).

Dizzy three times per week, lasting about five minutes. Head feels as if it is spinning inside. Objects do not move (1). Balance is better with fast walking (2).

Stress incontinence (2).

Back pain is worse with any motion; no pain if she does not move (2). Is worse now than after she fell in December.

Pain in the right arm has returned (1). "Cortisone must have worn off." Caused by impingement of her shoulder.

Sensation of constriction in her lower rib cage (1), "like a two-inch wide band."

Always hungry; eating huge amounts of food.

Desire for salt has diminished (1).

No lead-like feeling in her leg veins.

Slight fatigue, which goes away if she takes a short nap.

Bitter taste in mouth is gone.

Physical Examination:
- Weight: 152 lbs.
- Blood Pressure: 160/78.
- Pulse: 56 and regular.

Assessment: I reviewed the case for a moment. What do you think should have been done? I felt that the symptom picture was significantly changed. Angina was relatively minor now. The chest symptom was of a constrictive band in the lower part of the chest. Now, instead of borderline hypotension, her blood pressure was actually slightly high. She had marked constipation, ravenous hunger, amelioration from warm drinks, joint pain aggravated by even the slightest motion, and headaches from constipation. These symptoms clearly indicated Bryonia.

Plan: Bryonia 30c.

A Questionable Response to Bryonia

April 13, 1990

She told me that she felt better, with improvement of all of her minor symptoms except, oddly, her characteristically Bryonia back pain. Also, her angina was a bit worse. Now she was needing one nitroglycerin every other day. I felt concerned over the increase in the angina. I also was slightly concerned because, in researching Spigelia, I had repeatedly read the words, "Compare Bryonia."

The similarity of Spigelia and Bryonia is quite striking. The only keynote that they do not share is Bryonia's amelioration from firm pressure. Bryonia tends toward more irritability and has the strong fear of poverty, which Spigelia is not known to possess. They do share constipation, ravenous hunger, intense thirst, headaches, vertigo, and stitching or tearing pains worse with even the slightest motion.

Return to the First Remedy

April 19, 1990

The patient called me. Since 2 a.m. she had taken eight nitroglycerin because of dull, constrictive chest pain associated with a jittery anxiety, dizziness even when she lay down, and a pounding heart beating at only 37 beats per minute. She said that the heart was "pounding so hard that I can count it by feeling my body shake with the pounding."

Her back pain was still horrible and her legs felt heavy again.

(Here is another quote from the original proving of Spigelia: "Unusually strong beat of the heart, so that he not infrequently hears the heart beating; the heart's beat can also be seen through the clothes.")

Plan: I told her to take Spigelia 1M.

April 20, 1990

The next day she reported by telephone, "I feel ever so much better. My head is clear again. My chest feels wonderful." The comment about her head clearing, although she hadn't complained of confusion previously, led me to realize that part of the explanation for her inability to more clearly express her symptoms early in the case was because her mind was not as clear as it was now. She recognized this as well. Confusion and forgetfulness are emphasized strongly in the provings of Spigelia.

Additionally, she found that her shoulder and back were better.

May 20, 1990

When I last saw her on May 20 she was doing well.

Concluding Remarks

It is quite rewarding for me and my patient that homeopathic treatment has been able to effectively manage her organic heart disease.

Naturally, I wonder whether the arthritis of the knees, which led to the knee replacements, might have been cured by earlier treatment with Spigelia. I really believe her arthritis could have been prevented. Clarke found that the knees are specifically affected by Spigelia. He reported a couple of cases of people whose knee pain was cured with Spigelia. It's interesting in this case because her joint pathology has been overwhelmingly focused on her knees. The patient's other joints are not much affected, yet she has had surgery to replace both knees. I also wonder whether the prosthetic surgery and its complications might be obstacles to a permanent cure in this case.

Perhaps this patient might have been spared the April relapse if she had been the homeopath on the case, because she confided to me that when I gave her Bryonia she was thinking she should have more of the Spigelia. This is further proof of the innate wisdom of the patient.

Teresa Salvadore, DC

A CASE OF
WARTS & SLOW
MENTAL/EMOTIONAL
DEVELOPMENT

Teresa Salvadore, DC, has been a practicing chiropractor for eight years in Aspen, Colorado, and has studied homeopathy for seven years. She attended Miami University of Ohio and graduated from Logan College of Chiropractic in 1982. Teresa completed the IFH Professional Course in 1988 and has spent ten weeks of course study with George Vithoulkas. She is treasurer and a founding member of the National Board of Homeopathic Examiners. Teresa is also an instructor for the Texas Chiropractic College's post-graduate course in classical homeopathy.

The Patient Shows Signs of Mild Autism

Initial Visit: November 8, 1988

The patient was a five-year-old boy, who had been treated previously with Bryonia and Chamomilla for acute problems only.

Family History:
- Both great-grandfathers: alcoholism.
- Maternal grandfather: diabetes.
- Maternal grandmother: glaucoma.
- Paternal grandparents: alcoholism.
- Parents: healthy.

The patient was brought in for warts that appeared three weeks ago. He has plantar warts bilaterally, which are slightly inflamed, and one wart on his face. He never had problems with warts before. His only other skin complaint is a nonirritating perioral redness that has come and gone over the past several years.

The mother said he has problems with sleeplessness (2). He is very wakeful at night, but once he falls asleep he is usually fine. However, he had been awake from 1:30 to 4:30 a.m. a few nights previously, and wanted to get up and play. He usually sleeps on his stomach and thrashes around (2).

He hasn't been eating well recently. He usually craves dairy, especially yogurt (2), sweets (2), and Cheerios (2). He has an aversion to vegetables. He is thirsty for lukewarm water.

The mother described the child as strong-willed (2), but flexible. He gets fussy easily, whines, and cries if he has to take a nap. He is the "reluctant dragon," does not want to go to school, and likes a pacifier.

He is "a little behind": doesn't really write or draw yet, except for Os and Xs. He doesn't color, but he loves playing games and dot-to-dot.

The mother is concerned because he is so shy (2); if they have company, he is aware of them but doesn't interact with them.

He is very neat (3), cleans his room unsolicited, and wants to wash and change his clothes frequently. If anything gets on his hands, he will want to wash them (2), even leaving the dinner table in the middle of a meal. The mother said he was never trained to do this; in fact, the rest of the family is more on the messy side. His washing is a "joke around the house."

He has fears of being alone (3), follows his mother around the house, and is terrified if she goes outside without him. Sometimes he seems fearful in general, and the mother cannot pinpoint what he is afraid of. When sick, the child is afraid of the dark (2) and wants his hand held.

He has problems focusing mentally, especially when the family travels to an unfamiliar area.

The child gets hot easily (2), sticks his feet out of the covers (2), and perspires on his head (2).

Physical Examination:
- No salivation.
- Clear tongue.
- Strong, but short, teeth.

The child has a history of a heart murmur.

He is slightly constipated; takes longer to defecate than normal. He has no urinary problems. (His brother had problems with incontinence.)

No growing pains.

The child had surgery as an infant because he was born with webbed fingers. He also broke his collarbone while playing football, an injury that healed without complications.

(During the interview, the child hid under the examining table, would not look at me, and occasionally hit his mother while she was talking about him. The child has never been evaluated by a psychologist or psychiatrist, but mild autistic traits can be seen in the inability to interact with company, compulsive hand washing, and difficulty adjusting to any new environment.)

Case Analysis

When I was studying this case, I felt the center of gravity was on the mental plane, because of the rather extreme backwardness and the compulsive hand washing. This is a normal, straightforward family. They live in the country and are not neurotic in any apparent way. Therefore, the child's development of this compulsive habit was striking.

The remedy best known for compulsive hand washing is Syphilinum; additions from Barthel's *Synthetic Repertory* and from Vithoulkas are Coca, Lac caninum (2), Medorrhinum (2), Psorinum, and Natrum muriaticum. There are some indications for Medorrhinum, such as the desire for yogurt, the warts, sticking his feet out of the covers, and the fear of the dark. However, because of the backwardness of the child, his marked inability to interact with society, the history of deformities in his hands, and his short teeth, Syphilinum 1M was chosen.

It is interesting to note the relative absence of Syphilinum in Kent's repertory. We are all familiar with the night sufferings of Syphilinum; yet it is not listed under GENERALITIES, aggravated at night and pains at night, or MIND, fear at night. Although this was not a strong symptom in this case, it is a very strong symptom of the remedy and should be added to the repertory.

Boger, Clarke, and Allen mention the irritable and cross state of Syphilinum: "He does not want to be soothed and is violent on being opposed." This describes the emotional state of this boy when sick; he was previously given Bryonia and Chamomilla for acute states. Syphilinum can be found under "irritability with headaches" (in the highest degree) but not under "general irritability." Nor is Syphilinum listed for imbecility, insanity, obstinacy, or timidity, but all these traits are mentioned in the various materia medicas.

Concerning the insanity, we can look at the disease of syphilis. Boyd's textbook on pathology states that "Until recently syphilis was one of the common and important diseases in the world and was responsible for ten percent of all cases of insanity." It would be interesting to know the percentage of insanity that is caused by the syphilitic miasm. Boyd says that the syphilis seems to have lost its virulence ever since it was introduced to Europe by sailors returning with Christopher Columbus from the New World. He also states that it's the most subtle of all diseases. There's no syndrome for which it cannot be responsible, no symptomatology. And the more I study Syphilinum, the more I believe it is a subtle remedy. We need to be more alert to the possibility of using this remedy in our practices.

Another strong point for Syphilinum in this case is that it is one of the main remedies for the hereditary tendency to alcoholism. I discovered later that the child's father is a recovering alcoholic. Other remedies noted for hereditary alcoholism are Asarum, Tuberculinum, Psorinum, Sulphur, and Sulphuric acid.

When Vithoulkas talks about Syphilinum, he mentions the strong anxieties. They have fears, but they don't know what they are afraid of. We see this symptom in this case. The mother cannot pinpoint the child's fears. Syphilinum can be superstitious along with the hand washing, although I think this child is probably too young to manifest this superstition in any clear way.

Plan: Syphilinum 1M.

Syphilinum Helps on All Levels

Phone Consultation: November 23, 1988

The mother called and said the patient was doing really well. He was actually playing alone. The mother said she didn't realize the remedy could affect him emotionally, and said she felt free for the first time from his constant hanging on to her. However, the last few days he was a little anxious again.

The wart on his foot was less inflamed but still large.

He was sleeping better now, even during the full moon.

(The mother had not mentioned his difficulty with sleeping during the full moon at the initial interview. In "mental and general aggravation from moonlight," Antimonium crudum, Belladonna, and Thuja are found. Additions from Vithoulkas include Alumina, Calcarea carbonica, Causticum, Graphites, Sabadilla, and Silicea. From Boger, we can add, "aggravated every alternate full moon — Syphilinum.")

Assessment: This was the correct remedy. Definite amelioration can be seen on the mental and emotional planes.

Plan: Wait

A Minor Relapse from a Brief Illness

Phone Consultation: December 16, 1988

Progress on the warts had stopped. They were becoming painful, especially on his feet. He was anxious and constantly checking to see where his mother was. His sleep was good, sleeping until 5:30 a.m. every day. He was not waking at night, not washing his hands, but was constantly around his mother again: "Tell me where you are going."

He was becoming sensitive to touch on his collarbone, which he had broken. His mother stated that, when he had broken his collarbone and when he had the hand surgery, he didn't seem to be in pain, an almost abnormal underreaction.

Assessment: He had experienced a minor relapse, with fears and old symptoms returning.

Plan: Syphilinum 1M was given to hold and his mother was told to give it only if symptoms worsened and persisted.

Phone Consultation: December 28, 1988

He was never given the last remedy. He developed laryngitis, swollen tonsils, and congestion, but no pain. He had a fever, but it is gone now. Before this started, he was gray, listless, and couldn't talk, but he is fine now. He can play alone and seems to be recovering well from his illness.

Assessment: The minor relapse was due to an acute illness coming on. The patient improved on his own.

Plan: Wait.

New Eruptions Resemble Secondary Syphilis

Phone Consultation: January 4, 1989

The mother called to say that she and the patient's brother had recently recovered from strep throat. The whole family was put on antibiotics shortly after she last talked with me. After completing the antibiotics, a rash developed on the patient's abdomen and groin area, but it didn't seem to irritate him.

Plan: I advised them to wait because the rash was a possible allergic reaction to antibiotics and would probably go away.

January 17, 1989

The mother brought the patient in because the rash never went away. The eruption consisted of macular patches that became inflamed and, in the genital area, were somewhat ulcerated and scabbed. The lesions had traveled up the side of the neck to the hairline, lips, and around the mouth. There were no lesions inside the mouth, nose, or eyes, or elsewhere on the face. There were patches on the extremities, palms, and soles. The eruptions did not itch, but the mother was very concerned about the "angry" eruption around the genital region.

Mentally and emotionally, the patient was doing well. He was wanting to write, and was doing fine being alone. The mother noted that he was looking others directly in the eyes, talking, and communicating well. He was acting "less babyish." He was not washing his hands; in fact, he was almost too sloppy. The patient was very cooperative in showing me the lesions. He opened his mouth for me and did not hide or run away from me.

Assessment: Various eruptions can be produced by drug allergy; among these are urticaria, erythema nodosom and exfoliative dermatitis, as well as acneiform, mucocutaneous, lichenoid, and maculopapular types. (Maculopapular describes this boy's rash best.)

This boy's eruption was strikingly characteristic of secondary syphilis. In secondary syphilis, the eruption only mildly involves the trunk; it is more predominant on the genitalia and mucous membranes; and it pathognomonically affects the palms and soles. Secondary syphilis varies from faint, barely visible roseola to very prominent papular or plaque-like lesions. (The *Merck Manual* and Pillsbury and Heaton's *A Manual of Dermatology* were consulted.) The lesions may be transitory or may persist for months.

I felt strongly that the antibiotic had disturbed the case and helped to bring on a relapse, but it was not to the original symptomatic state of the case. The symptoms had seemingly gone from tertiary to secondary syphilitic symptoms. Interestingly, the boy had never had this before in his life. So, if we were "retracing symptoms," this could in some way be construed as a reversal of symptoms in past generations.

At this point in the case, I was at a loss. I first informed the mother as to what this eruption could be. Having seen the dramatic improvement on the mental and emotional plane, she was willing to do whatever was necessary to ensure progress in the case. Then Nick Nossaman, MD, pediatrician and homeopath, was consulted. He suggested blood work, such as the VDRL test, to screen for the possibility of syphilis. Because of the amelioration on the mental and emotional plane, he suggested waiting before repeating the remedy.

In spite of my insistence that blood work be done, the mother did not want to traumatize the boy emotionally by sticking him with needles. She felt that he had already gone through enough with his hand surgery and collarbone fracture. She was perfectly willing to wait out this eruption and, in that respect, was an ideal homeopathic follower. However, we will never be able to definitively identify this rash, because the blood work was not done.

Plan: Wait.

Occurrence of Pain from Previous Surgery

Phone Consultation: January 31, 1989

The patient was sleeping a lot, up to 14 hours. On Saturday night, he was crying and moaning, and didn't sleep until 4 a.m. The mother stated it was almost like he was going through surgery and expressing the pain (which he apparently had not felt when he went through the actual surgery).

The rash is better; it is moving down the body and leaving the head and upper extremities.

He is interested in learning and communicating; he is fine being alone.

Assessment: The patient is improving. Old symptoms are reappearing, and the eruption is leaving from above downward. It is interesting that the boy seemed to have "painlessness of complaints usually painful" (Helleborus, Opium, and Stramonium), but I was unable to find that symptom listed for Syphilinum in any of our materia medicas. It would be interesting to know if anyone else has seen that peculiarity in Syphilinum.

Plan: Wait.

Continued Improvement on Syphilinum

March 7, 1989

The wart on the right foot never went away and had been aggravated the last two weeks when the patient was skiing. The eruption has been coming and going; it was around the mouth the previous week, and the eruption in the groin area bled when he scratched it two days ago.

He has had his fingers in his mouth all the time for the past two weeks (an old habit when younger; would leave them in his mouth for hours).

He has been "very present with us." He has been interacting well with others.

No hand washing symptoms.

He has done a 180-degree turn in school; he is doing really well. He drew a self-portrait, which he had never attempted before. He is in preschool three full days. (His mother had withheld him from kindergarten because he wasn't ready.) His grandparents noted that he is finally affectionate and responding to them. Even his barber noted that he had really changed and "come out of his shell."

His mother thought that his teeth had grown.

Lately he was a little more tired than usual. He didn't want to go outside to play, and was better being alone, playing videos and games.

There were no other outstanding symptoms.

Assessment: The patient is doing well.

Plan: Wait.

Phone Consultation: March 14, 1989

The patient was up last night with an earache. He had a cold for three days, and coughed with a little bloody expectoration. He was "freaking" with the pain, shaking his head, and was awake with the pain from 9 p.m. to 4 a.m. Now, he was pale and not talking, and his ear no longer hurt. He had a fever the night before, with chills, a hot head, and perspiration on the head.

His breath had been bad since the cold started, and his thirst had increased.

He had eruptions on his arms.

There were no other remarkable symptoms.

Assessment: Acute ear inflammation.

Plan: Because the family lived some distance from the office, a remedy that the mother already had and that seemed to fit the symptoms was suggested in case the pain returned. The remedy was Mercurius vivus 30c.

April 11, 1989

The patient never used the Mercurius vivus. He was fine after the one episode of ear pain.

The eruptions are almost gone (three months after they began).

The wart on the foot persisted. The father was tired of waiting for the remedies to take care of it, and he threatened to call the dermatologist and have it burned off the next day. The child heard this, promptly went to his room, and picked it off. The wart has not returned to this day.

Another Dose of Syphilinum for a Mild Relapse

September 18, 1989

The child is in kindergarten now. His teacher says he is doing well at school.

No hand washing symptoms.

His throat has been bothering him; he has pain on coughing or before going to sleep (2). The coughing is worse during the later part of the day and at night (3). He has itching at the back of the throat (2).

He wants cold drinks (2), yogurt (2), and kefir (2).

He has a slight fever. His head is a little warm, but no perspiration. Tired (2) and chilly (2).

He wet his bed recently and has been up at night with bad dreams. He has been waking more frequently in general since school started. When he wakes at night he crawls into bed with his parents.

He has been irritable (2), grouchy (2), and back to some of his old patterns. He is fearful (2), quiet (2), and checking where his mother is all the time.

The child's lips were puffy (2) and red, but no perioral redness.

He has been drooling in his sleep.

No temper.

His eyes are red and watery.

Assessment: At this point, I felt the case had relapsed. We see his old behavioral patterns re-emerging, perhaps from the stress at school. It is not as severe as the initial visit, but we are seeing symptoms occurring at night.

Plan: Repeat Syphilinum 1M.

September 25, 1989

The patient has been fine. His disposition is better. His mother went away on a weekend trip, and he was fine.

March 1990

I contacted the mother, and she said that, in spite of family difficulties, the patient was doing very well in all aspects: mentally, emotionally, and physically. He has not needed any further doses of Syphilinum.

> *Peggy Chipkin: I used Syphilinum to treat a young girl about six or seven years old who could not stop washing her hands. She had tremendous anxiety about germs and touching things. It reached a peak when she was in the shower crying for her mother because every time she put the soap down she felt she had to pick it up and wash her hands again. About one or two weeks after she took the remedy, she experienced an aggravation of this symptom. Gradually the symptoms resolved, but it took several months for this problem to completely clear up.*
>
> *Salvadore: Thank you for sharing that. It's always good to hear another prescriber's experience.*

Frederik Schroyens, MD

SEVERAL CASES
OF
PNEUMONIA

Frederik Schroyens, MD, is a 1977 medical graduate of the State University of Ghent, Belgium, and a 1978 graduate of the one-year homeopathic training course at the Faculty for Homeopathy, London, England. Since 1981, Frederik has been the constitutive and continuing president of VSU, the largest and best-known school for homeopathic training in Belgium. He is also the constitutive president of the Masi Workshops in Belgium and Holland, has been homeopathic coordinator of the RADAR Project since 1986, and is a consultant for the Vithoulkas Expert System.

Introduction

In my country, we frequently have the opportunity to treat patients with pneumonia. Today, I will present seven pneumonia cases from my practice. Each of these cases will show you something different, either an instructive aspect of a commonly used remedy or the picture of an unusual remedy. I will emphasize the evaluation and assessment of each case, to show you different ways to approach a case. Once you have read and grasped the symptoms, then you must try to understand what is striking and characteristic about the case. This is how you can discover the true homeopathic symptoms and then translate them into rubrics, the language of the repertory.

Case Number 1

Female, Age 32

Initial Interview: November 21, 1989

She has pain in the left upper chest, near the shoulder. Yesterday, it extended into the shoulder.

A sudden onset, with a fever of 39°C (102.2°F).

The pain is much worse when she is lying on her left side (3); cannot breathe.

Her chest is painful when she coughs (2) and when she breathes in (2).

She has pain in both ears, especially the right one; worse when she eructates and coughs.

Frequent eructations.

She has pain in the chest from eructations (2) and laughing (2).

A kind of nausea occurs when she coughs.

When the pain becomes worse, it extends from the region of the left shoulder to the stomach.

The chest is aggravated as soon as she lies down, but especially when lying on the left side.

She has been dizzy since yesterday evening (onset of fever).

She has a pain in her stomach from coughing, and she retches from the pain.

She is generally very pale, looks exhausted and sick.

For the past week, she has not felt "like usual." Has been tired with a sore throat.

She weeps more easily.

Is not hungry at all, although she has a very empty feeling in the stomach.

She likes to be in the living room, to be with people, but quietly.

Analysis of Case Number 1

The choice is between Bryonia and Phosphorus. They both cover the general elements. At first glance, one might not prescribe Bryonia, because of its well-known keynote of amelioration from pressure (this patient is aggravated by lying on the painful side). It is good to know the general picture of a remedy and its keynotes, but it is also good to look for exceptions. Note that Bryonia is listed in the repertory, albeit in lesser degree, for chest pain aggravated by lying on the painful side. So, this is an exception for Bryonia.

In order to further differentiate between these two remedies, I did what is called a comparative extraction, using the RADAR computer program (from ARCHIBEL). This allowed for a more detailed search through the CHEST section of the repertory, comparing only Bryonia and Phosphorus. I often do this to develop clear-cut and very precise pictures of remedies. In this case, the comparative extraction made it very clear that Bryonia is much stronger for the right side of the chest, while Phosphorus is

			No. of remedies in the rubric
S-v2.2	1234 3	1 a CHEST. - PAIN - lying,while - side,on - affected	4
S-v2.2	1234 3	2 a CHEST. - PAIN - lying,while - side,on - painful	5
S-v2.2	1234 3	3 a CHEST. - PAIN - Sides - lying, - on left side - painful side - agg.	4
S-v2.2	1234 3	4 a CHEST. - PAIN - sore,bruised - Sides - left - lying on painful side	1
S-v2.2	1234 3	5 a CHEST. - PAIN - stitching - lying, - side, - on the affected	3
S-v2.2	1234 3	6 a CHEST. - PAIN - stitching - lying, - side, - on the painful	2
S-v2.2	1234 3	7 a CHEST. - PAIN - stitching - Sides - left - lying - on left side agg.	6
S-v2.2	1234 2	8 - CHEST. - PAIN - eructation, - from	3
S-v2.2	1234 1	9 - EAR - PAIN - eructations,during	2
S-v2.2	1234 2	10 - CHEST. - PAIN - Sides - cough,during	30
S-v2.2	1234 2	11 - CHEST. - PAIN - Sides - inspiration	44
S-v2.2	1234 2	12 - VERTIGO - HEAT, - during the	21
S-v2.2	1234 1	13 - STOMACH - PAIN - coughing,from	35
S-v2.2	1234 2	14 - COUGH. - LAUGHING	27
S-v2.2	1234 2	15 - CHEST. - PAIN - laughing	5
S-v2.2	1234 1	16 - STOMACH - EMPTINESS - hunger,without	27
S-v2.2	1234 2	17 - CHEST. - PAIN - Sides - left	58

	1 phos.	2 bry.	3 kali-c.	4 rumx.	5 lyc.	6 rhus-t.	7 ars.	7 sil.	9 ran-b.	10 sep.	11 cocc.	12 bell.	13 stann.	13 sulph.
	8[a]/14[b]	7/13	4/7	4/8	4/7	5/7	5/6	5/6	3/7	4/6	4/5	3/6	3/7	4/8
	[c]15/27	13/23	9/16	8/17	8/13	8/10	8/9	8/9	7/16	7/10	7/9	6/14	6/13	6/13
1a	-	-	-	-	-	-	-	-	-	-	-	2	-	-
2a	-	1	-	1	-	-	-	-	2	-	-	3	-	-
3a	-	-	-	2	-	-	-	-	2	-	-	2	-	-
4a	-	-	-	2	-	-	-	-	-	-	-	-	-	-
5a	-	-	2	-	-	-	-	-	-	-	-	-	-	-
6a	-	-	-	-	-	-	-	-	-	-	-	-	1	-
7a	2	-	-	2	2	-	-	-	-	-	-	-	2	-
8-	1	-	-	-	-	-	-	-	-	-	1	-	-	-
9-	-	-	-	-	-	-	-	-	-	-	-	-	-	1
10-	2	3	-	-	1	1	1	-	-	2	-	2	-	3
11-	-	3	2	3	1	-	1	1	2	1	1	-	-	-
12-	1	1	2	-	-	-	-	-	-	1	2	-	-	-
13-	2	3	-	1	3	2	2	1	-	2	-	1	3	-
14-	2	1	1	-	-	1	1	1	-	-	-	-	2	-
15-	-	-	-	-	-	-	-	-	-	-	-	-	-	-
16-	1	1	-	-	-	2	1	2	-	-	1	-	-	2
17-	3	-	-	2	-	1	-	1	3	-	-	-	-	2

[a] No. of rubrics covered by the remedy.
[b] Total score, based on whether the remedy is plain, italic or bold in each rubric.
[c] Alternative score, taking intensity of the symptom in the case into account.

equally strong for the left side. This was enough for me to make the choice for Phosphorus as the prescription.

The same symptoms analyzed with the Vithoulkas Expert System (also from ARCHIBEL) show the following result:

```
-------------------------------------------HELP IN PRESCRIBING-------------------------------------------
|                                                                                                       |
| So far the best probability is phos. 115.5ᵃ (confidence rating 118 pts)                               |
|                                                                                                       |
-------------------------------------------HELP IN INTERROGATION-----------------------------------------
|                                                                                                       |
|                                                                                                       |
---------------------------------------------------------------------------------------------------------
```

	This analysis contains 17 single symptoms and compares patterns of 138 remedies	phos.		
1 a CHEST. - PAIN - lying,while - side,on - affected				
1 a CHEST. - PAIN - lying,while - side,on - painful				
1 a CHEST. - PAIN - Sides - lying, - on left side - painful side - agg.				
1 a CHEST. - PAIN - sore,bruised - Sides - left - lying on painful side				
1 a CHEST. - PAIN - stitching - lying, - side, - on the affected				
1 a CHEST. - PAIN - stitching - lying, - side, - on the painful				
1 a CHEST. - PAIN - stitching - Sides - left - lying - on left side agg.		3[b]	2[c]	14[d]
2 CHEST. - PAIN - eructation, - from		2	1	3
3 EAR - PAIN - eructations,during		1	-	2
4 CHEST. - PAIN - Sides - cough,during		2	2	30
5 CHEST. - PAIN - Sides - inspiration		2	-	44
6 VERTIGO - HEAT, - during the		2	1	21
7 STOMACH - PAIN - coughing,from		1	2	35
8 COUGH. - LAUGHING		2	2	27
9 CHEST. - PAIN - laughing		2	-	5
10 STOMACH - EMPTINESS,weak feeling,faintness,goneness,hungry feeling - hunger,without		1	1	27
11 CHEST. - PAIN - Sides - left		2	3	58

[a] Absolute score, should be greater than 100 to give confidence in the remedy suggested. If it is greater than 100, fewer possible remedies are suggested, thereby narrowing the field of likely remedies to consider for the case.
[b] Intensity of the symptom in the case.
[c] Degree of the remedy in the repertory.
[d] Size of the rubric in the repertory.

The Vithoulkas Expert System (VES) analysis comes up strongly for one remedy, which is again Phosphorus. Thus, Phosphorus was prescribed with a considerable degree of confidence.

Plan: Phosphorus 200c, one dose every two hours until a reaction occurs.

Follow-Up on Case Number 1

She took the remedy in the early afternoon. That night she could lie down, but she still had a lot of pain in the chest. The fever was still present.

Day 1:   The next morning she had some appetite and ate a little bit.

Plan: Stop regular intake of the remedy.

During that day, she felt the pain diminishing steadily. She coughed a lot, but it was less painful. By the evening, the fever was almost gone. She still felt very weak.

Plan: No remedy.

Day 2:   Her weakness persisted. Her appetite returned. The pains and fever have almost disappeared. She is breathing more easily. She still complains about the pain in her ears.

Plan: No remedy.

Day 3:   The pulmonary symptoms are now only in the background. She is still expectorating and coughing. The pain in the ears is worse; it can persist for several hours and then go away for a while.

Plan: No remedy.

Day 4:   She is the same as before. Her ears are very painful.

Plan: Phosphorus 1M, one dose.

Day 5: All symptoms have disappeared.

Jacqueline Wilson: What did the ears look like on examination?

Schroyens: The exam was normal, no inflammation. So, when a remedy has produced improvement, we do not like to go away from it. I therefore gave a dose of Phosphorus 1M. The pain in the ears vanished within a few hours, and she made a complete recovery.

Audience: How many doses of the Phosphorus 200c did she take?

Schroyens: She started the remedy at 1 or 2 p.m. and then took it every two hours throughout the night. When I spoke with her the next morning, I felt that her ability to lie down more easily and her slightly improved appetite were sufficient indications to tell her to stop the remedy, because the case was moving in a positive direction.

Case Number 2

Female, Age 34

Initial Interview: February 8, 1989

She has had pneumonia for the last ten days. She started with antibiotics (Cefadroxil and Duracef) but had no clear reaction, except that the fever disappeared. Another stronger antibiotic was started, but she reacted to it with repeated vomiting. Cefadroxil was then started again, at the maximum dose. Because there was still no reaction, hospitalization was recommended. She came to see me to try to avoid hospitalization.

She is very, very weak; walks in step by step, leaning on her husband's shoulder. She moves very slowly. She can barely speak; there is no power in her voice.

She still has a fever; 37.5°C (99.5°F) today.

Her ears feel closed by some pressure (for four days); she doesn't hear herself speaking.

She can barely breathe, speaks in whispers, avoids any respiration movements, pants slowly.

She has been sweating profusely at night. She had to change her nightgown three times last night.

Her skin is pale and shows some type of soft red-blue network, which is especially pronounced on the lower extremities and knees.

She is afraid to be alone. She believes she is going to die. She feels that at any moment she could suffocate and that she has to concentrate on how to breathe.

(She begins to cry silently.)

Her cough is worse at night. Regular paroxysms begin at about 4 p.m. and diminish at 4 a.m., after which she falls asleep.

She feels restless during the night and has confused dreams.

She has no hunger.

Her difficulty in breathing is aggravated by the coughing and by tobacco smoke.

She is constipated.

When the fever was higher (40°C, or 104°F), she imagined that she heard thieves in the house.

She wants her husband to be with her and to talk to her.

Desires cold drinks, really cold, from the refrigerator.

During the pneumonia she had already received eight remedies, without effect:

- Arsenicum album
- Aconitum
- Belladonna
- China
- Bryonia
- Carbo vegetabilis

- Phosphorus
- Sepia

Analysis of Case Number 2

				No. of remedies in the rubric
S-v2.2	1234 2	1 - EAR - STOPPED sensation		116
S-v2.2	1234 4	2 - GENERAL - WEAKNESS,enervation		659
S-v2.2	1234 3	3 - PERSPIRATION. - PROFUSE - night		64
S-v2.2	1234 1	4 a EXTREMITIES. - DISCOLORATION, - Lower Limbs, - marbled		3
S-v2.2	1234 1	5 a EXTREMITIES. - DISCOLORATION, - Thigh, - marbled		1
S-v2.2	1234 1	6 a EXTREMITIES. - DISCOLORATION, - Leg, - marbled		1
S-v2.2	1234 2	7 - MIND - FEAR,apprehension,dread - alone,of being		50
S-v2.2	1234 1	8 - MIND - RESTLESSNESS - night		244
S-v2.2	1234 1	9 - GENERAL - AFTERNOON(13-18h) - 16-4h		1
S-v2.2	1234 1	10 - DREAMS - CONFUSED		122
S-v2.2	1234 1	11 - MIND - DELUSIONS - thieves, - house,in		9
S-v2.2	1234 2	12 - GENERAL - FOOD and DRINKS - cold drink,cold water - desire		129

	1	2	3	4	4	6	7	7	7	10	11	12
	lyc.	phos.	merc.	ars.	verat.	arg-n.	bry.	nat-c.	thuj.	nat-m.	caust.	sulph.
	$8^a/18^b$	7/17	7/17	7/14	7/13	7/13	7/12	7/12	8/12	7/12	7/14	6/14
	$^c16/36$	15/40	15/39	15/32	15/32	15/28	15/27	15/27	15/27	14/27	14/26	13/32
1-	3	2	3	1	2	2	1	2	1	1	2	2
2-	2	3	3	3	3	2	2	2	2	3	2	3
3-	2	3	3	2	2	1	2	2	3	2	1	3
4a	1	-	-	-	-	-	-	-	1	-	3	-
5a	-	-	-	-	-	-	-	-	-	-	3	-
6a	-	-	-	-	-	-	-	-	-	-	3	-
7-	3	3	1	3	1	3	1	1	-	-	-	-
8-	3	2	3	3	1	2	1	1	1	1	3	3
9-	-	-	-	-	-	-	-	-	1	-	-	-
10-	2	1	-	-	1	1	2	2	1	2	1	2
11-	-	-	1	1	-	-	-	-	-	2	-	-
12-	2	3	3	1	3	2	3	2	2	1	2	1

[a] No. of rubrics covered by the remedy.
[b] Total score, based on whether the remedy is plain, italic or bold in each rubric.
[c] Alternative score, taking intensity of the symptom in the case into account.

No one remedy is clearly indicated. The VES also does not suggest a remedy for prescription, but, surprisingly, puts Thuja as a first possibility to consider:

SMALL REMEDIES		MEDIUM REMEDIES		LARGE REMEDIES	
kali-fcy.	****	cupr-a.	*****	thuj.	**********
agar-ph.	***	arist-cl.	*****	arg-n.	*********
digox.	***	sol-t-ae.	****	kali-p.	*******
zinc-ar.	***	ars-s-f.	****	clem.	*******
bals-p.	***	merc-cy.	****	verat.	*******
mom-b.	***	aur-ar.	****	ars.	*******
nat-sal.	***	calc-ar.	****	ant-t.	******
antip.	***	nat-hchls.	****	lyc.	******
irid.	*	bol-la.	***	nat-p.	******
zinc-pic.	*	digin.	***	merc.	******
spirae.	*	lec.	***	phos.	******
ant-ar.	*	calc-i.	***	bism.	******
sarcol-ac.	*	echi.	***	nat-c.	******
aven.	*	ferr-m.	***	nit-ac.	******
kiss.	*	cadm-s.	***	kali-c.	*****
lol.	*	anag.	***	apis	*****
menis.	*	nat-ar.	***	con.	*****
agar-em.	*	alet.	***	camph.	*****
ben.	*	hydrc.	***	sil.	*****
ven-m.	*	merc-sul.	***	bry.	*****

So, I began to reflect on Thuja. Do you know what Thuja is? Thuja occidentalis is the "tree of life." It is a very big, impressive tree. This is probably why it has such a name, because it was thought to demonstrate so clearly the idea of strength and the energy of growth. And, as you know, we homeopaths use Thuja to treat all kinds of growths — warts, tumors, fibroids. What is equally interesting about Thuja is that it contains another aspect in its symptomatology that contradicts this idea of life and strength. This is the aspect of weakness, fragility, division, and death. It is a special fragility, a feebleness. Thuja makes a bridge between life and death, between strength and weakness, and between power and fragility. Both sides are encompassed in its materia medica.

The following is a list of some of Thuja's delusions that demonstrate this aspect:

Page	Symptoms	DEG[a]	LGTH[b]
1	MIND - DELUSIONS,imaginations,hallucinations,illusions	0	190
1	MIND - DELUSIONS, - body, - brittle,is	1	1
1	MIND - DELUSIONS, - body, - delicate,is - - - - - - - - - - - - - - -	2	1
1	MIND - DELUSIONS, - body, - lighter than air,is	1	5
1	MIND - DELUSIONS, - body, - pieces,in danger of coming in	1	1
1	MIND - DELUSIONS, - body, - thin,is	1	1
1	MIND - DELUSIONS, - die, - he was about to - - - - - - - - - - -	2	27
1	MIND - DELUSIONS, - die, - time has come to	1	5
1	MIND - DELUSIONS, - diminished, - thin,he is too	1	1
1	MIND - DELUSIONS, - divided into two parts	1	9
1	MIND - DELUSIONS, - divided into two parts - cut in two parts, or - which part he had possession on waking,and could not tell of	1	1
1	MIND - DELUSIONS, - double, - of being	1	30
1	MIND - DELUSIONS, - emaciation, of	1	4
1	MIND - DELUSIONS, - glass, - she is made of	1	1
1	MIND - DELUSIONS, - glass, - wood,glass,etc.being made of - -	2	3
1	MIND - DELUSIONS, - head - belongs to another	1	6
1	MIND - DELUSIONS, - heavy,is	1	2
1	MIND - DELUSIONS, - light, - incorporeal,he is	1	16
1	MIND - DELUSIONS, - pregnant, she is	1	12

[a] Degree of the remedy in the repertory — whether it is plain (1), italic (2), or bold (3).
[b] Length of the rubric in the repertory.

You will not find very much information in our literature concerning Thuja and pneumonia. But this was a case where several of the more commonly used pneumonia remedies had already been tried. The weakness of this patient was quite striking. It was as though I were sitting in front of a corpse. It was a situation where death was not far away. In addition to the extreme weakness, there was another symptom to support Thuja: worse from 4 p.m. to 4 a.m. (this is a repertory addition from Stauffer, in which Thuja is the only remedy listed). So, I decided to prescribe Thuja.

Plan: Thuja 200c, one dose every two hours until a change occurs.

Follow-Up on Case Number 2

She took the remedy in my office and called back the next day.

Day 1: She woke up the previous night and was perspiring very profusely (as she had done the previous nights). She started having a very foul and copious discharge from the nose that kept her awake for several hours. She fell asleep again toward the morning.

The physician, who knew she was seeing a homeopath, called her. She laughed, telling him "I am cured!" The fever had fallen completely, and she had her first breakfast in a long time, with a good appetite.

Her reaction was probably a bit optimistic; she was still very weak, with labored respiration.

Plan: Stop repetition of the remedy.

Day 2: Her appetite had returned and her respiration was easier, but she was still very weak.

Plan: No remedy.

Day 3: She was coughing more. She felt desperate again. Weakness. Some slight fever. Very painful in the ribs.

Plan: Thuja 1M.

Day 4: Her respiration was better, but the pain in the chest continued to upset her quite a lot.

Plan: Repeat Thuja 1M.

Day 5: The pain in the ribs had become the main problem; all other symptoms had decreased significantly. It was apparent that this pain was mostly in the right short ribs. In the repertory, I found the following:

- CHEST: Pain, sore, short ribs, right (Chelidonium, Lycopodium).
- CHEST: Pain, inflammation of lungs, after (Lycopodium is bold type).

Plan: Lycopodium 200c, one dose. (Remember that Lycopodium was strongly represented in the initial computer analysis.)

Day 6: Her chest pain had diminished; the respiratory problems continued to decrease.

Plan: No remedy. A complete recovery ensued.

Additional Remarks on Case Number 2

- Also consider the following two rubrics (both for Thuja):

  - RESPIRATION: Difficult, sternum, from pressure on.
  - RESPIRATION: Impeded, stitches in chest.

- The copious elimination from her nose on the first night was a very good sign.

- Borland mentions that Lycopodium is a remedy that typically comes in at the second stage of pneumonia.

Case Number 3

Male, Age 1

Initial Interview: February 10, 1979

The illness began two days ago with a green discharge from the nose and with some rattling in the chest, which was heard especially when crying. The next day, the green discharge reappeared, along with green pus from the eyes. In the evening, a high fever suddenly set in. The night was all right, but this morning the baby is really sick. His fever is now 39.1°C (102.4°F). His eyes are closed from the discharge, he has a lot of greenish discharge from the nose, and his breathing is very difficult.

His stool is green, papescent, and sticks to the skin (2).

His urine has a bad odor.

He is thirsty (2).

His appetite diminishes quickly.

He doesn't cough when he is quiet, coughs a little when he is sleeping, and coughs more when he has been crying for a while (2).

Some swelling under the eyes.

Analysis of Case Number 3

			No. of remedies in the rubric
S-v2.2	1234 2	1 - NOSE - DISCHARGE, - greenish	68
S-v2.2	1234 1	2 - EYE - DISCHARGES - purulent	35
S-v2.2	1234 2	3 - STOOL. - FATTY,greasy	7
S-v2.2	1234 2	4 - STOOL. - GREEN	90
S-v2.2	1234 1	5 - URINE. - ODOR - offensive	91
S-v2.2	1234 2	6 - STOMACH - THIRST - heat, - during	79
S-v2.2	1234 2	7 - COUGH. - CRYING agg.	16
S-v2.2	1234 1	8 - FACE - SWELLING - eyes, - under	22

	1 phos.	2 sulph.	3 ars.	4 hep.	5 lyc.	6 puls.	7 sep.	8 calc.	9 nux-v.	10 colch.	11 merc.	12 cham.	13 arn.	13 bry.
	8^a/14^b	8/15	7/13	6/11	6/10	6/14	5/11	5/11	5/9	5/6	5/12	4/8	4/8	4/7
	^{c}13/24	13/23	12/21	10/18	10/15	9/22	8/17	8/16	8/15	8/9	7/18	7/14	7/13	7/13
1-	2	1	1	1	1	3	3	1	1	1	3	-	1	2
2-	1	2	-	3	3	3	2	3	-	-	3	2	-	-
3-	2	1	1	-	-	-	-	-	-	-	-	-	-	-
4-	3	3	2	2	2	3	2	2	2	1	3	3	-	1
5-	2	3	2	1	2	2	3	3	2	1	2	-	3	-
6-	2	2	3	2	1	2	1	2	3	1	-	2	1	3
7-	1	1	1	2	1	-	-	-	-	-	-	1	3	-
8-	1	2	3	-	-	1	-	-	1	2	1	-	-	1

[a] No. of rubrics covered by the remedy.
[b] Total score, based on whether the remedy is plain, italic or bold in each rubric.
[c] Alternative score, taking intensity of the symptom in the case into account.

The sudden appearance of the high fever in the evening is typical for many pneumonias — a sudden onset, a high fever, and a general state of collapse. The baby had the marked difficulty with breathing that is usual for pneumonia. The right lung was more affected. The computer analysis suggests Phosphorus and Sulphur. In deciding between them, I took into account some "intangible" aspects. This was a beautiful little baby, surrounded by a loving family. The baby was quiet and relatively content as long as he was close to his parents, brother, and sister. There was a feeling that the child was surrounded by affection and clearly seemed to need and attract this attention. It was this aspect that led me to choose Phosphorus over Sulphur. Also, note that the stickiness of the stool suggests some concomitant liver involvement (due to an increased fat content in the stool), which is another point in favor of Phosphorus.

Plan: Phosphorus 2/50M, one dose every hour. (I was using the LM potencies more at that time.)

Follow-Up on Case Number 3

At 7:30 p.m. on the day he took the remedy, he ate his normal amount of food.

Day 1, morning: He cried for three hours and coughed a lot, then slept 30 minutes, and again cried for a while. His urine and breath were very offensive. His fever was 38.2°C (100.8°F).

Plan: Continue remedy four times per day.

Day 1, evening: The child was brought in to see me. His fever was 38.7°C (101.7°F). His skin texture was normal again. One eye was agglutinated. Auscultation: all symptoms in the chest had vanished.

Plan: Continue the remedy four times per day.

Day 2, evening: The fever had not been more than 37.5°C (99.5°F) all day. The child was playing again.

Plan: Discontinue the remedy. He made a full recovery.

Additional Remarks on Case Number 3

Phosphorus is often indicated for young children. This particular case is not especially typical of the Phosphorus pneumonia, so I would like to mention some of the key symptoms that occur more routinely:

- Dry air passages, with a burning feeling.

- Great thirst, especially for cold water.

- Yellow and diarrheic stools, sometimes blood-streaked (liver problems).

- Often the lower half of the right lung is involved (also pain in the left chest, aggravated by lying on the left side).

- Expectoration of mucus with blood streaks.

- Desires company; fears being alone.

Also consider the following rubrics:

- GENERALITIES: Mucous secretions increased, greenish (Phosphorus is italics).

- RESPIRATION: Rattling (Phosphorus is bold type).

- NOSE: Discharge, crusts, green, masses (Phosphorus is italics).

Audience: Why did you continue to give the remedy when the child was improving?

Schroyens: Because at that time in my practice I was systematically using the LM potencies, and the rule in this approach is to continue administering the remedy, even after improvement has begun. As you probably know, this was described by Hahnemann in the later editions of the Organon.

Case Number 4

Male, Age 16 Months

Initial Interview: October 13, 1986

Bronchitis had set in on October 3. Two remedies were prescribed over the telephone. They were unsuccessful. The physician in charge told the parents that a pneumonia had set in and that antibiotics were absolutely necessary because the child's state had worsened considerably. Novabritine was given for one week, immediately reducing the fever but only slowly ameliorating the general symptoms. The day the antibiotics were stopped, the child grew worse within hours and his fever rose to 40°C (104°F) again.

He hasn't eaten much for several days; his thirst is moderate.

He is a very nice and lovely child. He caresses and holds his little puppet closely. He is also very nice to his brother.

He laughs when unimportant things happen and seems to be amused by what others do wrong.

Has laughed during his sleep for the past several nights.

He does not want his usual fruit compote; wants to eat what his parents eat (2).

Is afraid of noises, such as the vacuum cleaner; weeps.

Even though he laughs frequently when small things happen, he generally looks rather earnest, which is quite unusual for him.

Analysis of Case Number 4

```
-----------------------------------HELP IN PRESCRIBING-----------------------------------
|                                                                                        |
| So far the best probability is lyc. 378.3ᵃ (confidence rating 101 pts)                |
|                                                                                        |
-----------------------------------HELP IN INTERROGATION-----------------------------------
|                                                                                        |
| Also ask questions about                                                               |
|                                                                                        |
| puls.                                                                                  |
|                                                                                        |
```

	puls.	lyc.		
This analysis contains 14 single symptoms and compares patterns of 164 remedies				
1 FACE - DISCOLORATION, - pale - heat,during	1[b]	2[c]	1[d]	14[e]
2 MIND - MILDNESS	3	2	3	76
3 FEVER. - SLEEP,heat comes on - during	2	2	2	54
4 a MIND - LAUGHING - easily				
4 a MIND - LAUGHING - ludicrous,everything seems				
4 a MIND - LAUGHING - misfortune,at				
4 a MIND - LAUGHING - mocking				
4 a MIND - LAUGHING - trifles,at	2	2	2	16
5 MIND - LAUGHING - sleep,during	2	3	-	15
6 b MIND - FEAR,apprehension,dread - noise,from				
6 b MIND - STARTING,startled - noise,from				
6 b MIND - WEEPING,tearful mood - noise,at	2	2	-	70
7 MIND - ENVY	2	1	2	21
8 MIND - SERIOUS,earnest	2	1	1	63

[a] Absolute score (should be >100); if greater than 100, few Rxs suggested.
[b] Intensity of symptom in the case.
[c] Lyc. degree of remedy in the repertory for the indicated symptom.
[d] Puls. degree of remedy in the repertory for the indicated symptom.
[e] Size rubric.

What is initially striking in this case is the laughing. This symptom is not typical in a case of pneumonia, and it therefore qualifies as a "strange, rare, and peculiar" symptom. I interpreted his attitude toward food as envy — he wants what someone else has. And then there is the serious, earnest look on his face. These symptoms strongly suggest Lycopodium. Lycopodium was given, with very good results.

Plan: Lycopodium 200c, one dose.

Follow-Up on Case Number 4

After taking the remedy, he was restless that night. He cried a lot. He had a fever the whole night.

Day 1:   The child slept in the morning and woke up with only a slight fever. The fever increased again toward the evening. The cough diminished, and the child looked brighter and reacted more easily to contacts.

   Plan: No repetition of the remedy.

Day 2:   He was slightly better than the day before. Not much fever.

   Plan: No repetition of the remedy.

Day 3:   He was slightly better again. He slept through the night.

   Plan: No repetition of the remedy. A complete recovery ensued.

Additional Remarks on Case Number 4

The following are other typical symptoms for Lycopodium:

- Earnest, including frowning of the forehead.

- Fan-like motion of alae nasi.

- Very serious, unresolved conditions.

- Loud rales, yellow and thick expectoration.

- Coldness of the right foot, with fever in children.

- Flatulence, a little food fills up the stomach.

- Fever is worse between 4 and 8 p.m.

Discussion on the Earnestness of Lycopodium

I would like to describe the earnestness of Lycopodium as it applies to adults. Imagine a person sitting there, looking so earnest and serious. He's looking off into the distance. He's thinking, wondering, and worrying: "Will I get there? Will it work out?" In the repertory under the rubric — MIND, fear, of being unable to reach his destination — Lycopodium is the only remedy listed. This gives the feeling of a kind of uncertainty, a kind of worry.

And then, in the SLEEP section of the repertory, we find Lycopodium in the rubric — SLEEP, dreams, drowning in a foundering boat. He can't reach his destination because he's rowing in a foundering boat. He has good reason to look so serious.

There is a third aspect of Lycopodium. Imagine him in this boat, ordering others around. "All right, you men over there must do this, do that...and you over there, bring me that oar and be quick about it. The captain is coming soon, and we must be ready to follow his orders." He becomes dictatorial, intolerant to contradiction, hard on inferiors, and respectful of superiors in order to get the others involved and to reach his destination. He makes everyone run, because the captain is coming. The captain represents power, and Lycopodium loves power.

So, taking all of this together, we get an idea of how life is for Lycopodium. He takes life very seriously. He has a deep inner feeling of insecurity that affects everything he does. This is the earnestness of Lycopodium.

Case Number 5

Male, Age 22 Months

Initial Interview: November 24, 1989

He has had a fever of 39.2°C (102.6°F) since yesterday, and started coughing and having difficulty breathing.

He has one red cheek (2).

He doesn't sit anymore; he's been lying down since the onset of his illness.

He is very nervous. When playing, he gets irritated when the blocks in his game do not fit on each other.

Is not hungry, hasn't eaten since yesterday.

Has a very loose cough; you can hear the rattling (2).

Cold feet.

Didn't want to be left at his grandmother's place.

Wanted to eat some soup only if he could sit on his father's lap; wants to stay there.

Is angry and cross if he is forbidden something.

Is unusually thirsty, drinks one normal-sized glass in one stroke.

Analysis of Case Number 5

```
-------------------------------------------HELP IN PRESCRIBING------------------------------------------
|                                                                                               |
| So far the best probability is sulph. 409.9ᵃ (confidence rating 102 pts)                      |
|                                                                                               |
-------------------------------------------HELP IN INTERROGATION-----------------------------------------
|                                                                                               |
| Also ask questions about                                                                      |
|                                                                                               |
| ars.                                                                                          |
|                                                                                               |
--------------------------------------------------------------------------------------------------------
```

		ars	sulph.		
	This analysis contains 8 single symptoms and compares patterns of 133 remedies				
1	GENERAL - WEAKNESS,enervation - fever, - during	1ᵇ	1ᶜ	3ᵈ	5ᵉ
2 a	FACE - DISCOLORATION, - red - one-sided				
2 a	FACE - DISCOLORATION, - red - one-sided - one pale the other red	2	1	1	29
3	MIND - ANGER,irascibility - mistakes,about his	2	2	1	6
4	EXTREMITIES. - COLDNESS - Foot - fever,during	1	2	1	30
5	COUGH. - RATTLING	2	2	-	73
6	MIND - CARRIED,desires to be	2	1	2	29
7	STOMACH - THIRST - large quantities,for	3	3	3	27

ᵃ Absolute score (should be >100); if greater than 100, few Rxs suggested.
ᵇ Intensity of symptom in the case.
ᶜ Sulph.degree of remedy in the repertory for the indicated symptom.
ᵈ Ars.degree of remedy in the repertory for the indicated symptom.
ᵉ Size rubric.

The child developed pneumonia while staying at his grandmother's house. The grandmother had developed pneumonia a few days earlier and was still sick with it. She told her daughter, "Quick, get the doctor to prescribe antibiotics. I'm very sick, and I don't want my little grandchild to suffer in the same way." But the parents called the homeopath.

As you can see from the VES analysis, the case is strong for Sulphur. The red cheek, the thirst for large quantities, the cold feet during fever, and the weakness during fever suggest Sulphur. I interpreted the child's attitude toward the blocks as anger about his mistakes, which is also a Sulphur symptom. One important characteristic of the acute Sulphur picture is an uneven distribution of blood, of body temperature. One part is very hot, and another is quite cold. Often the lips are bright red during acute illnesses, or there is excess heat on top of the head. In this case, the feet were quite cold.

Plan: Sulphur 30c, one dose every 30 minutes until a change occurs.

Follow-Up on Case Number 5

Evening after the interview: The remedy was taken the same day at about 5 p.m. It was repeated two times that same evening. During the evening, he began sitting up again. By the time he went to bed, his temperature was 38.7°C (101.7°F). No other change.

Plan: Repeat the remedy once or twice today, then stop.

Day 1: All symptoms disappeared: No fever, he was eating again, and his usual, kind temperament had returned. His cough continued.

Plan: No remedy. Complete recovery followed. His grandmother was still sick and still taking antibiotics.

Additional Remarks on Case Number 5

The following are other typical symptoms for Sulphur:

- Especially the left lung.

- "Redness": face or lips.

- Heat: hot palms and/or soles; hot vertex.

- Many rales in the chest; mucopurulent expectoration; a lot going on in the chest.

- Coldness in one foot, especially the left one (Lycopodium, especially the right one — Farrington).

Case Number 6

Female, Age 5 1/2

Initial Interview: December 12, 1988

She has had a fever for two days; today, it is 39.5°C (103.1°F).

Her sleep is restless, with perspiration.

She cries and feels annoyed because of the perspiration.

She has a deep, very loose cough.

Increasing mental restlessness.

She has some coryza and has definite pain in the ear when she blows her nose.

She asks for a drink when she wakes at night.

She weeps easily, looks unhappy, and cannot bear to be contradicted.

Analysis of Case Number 6

			No. of remedies in the rubric
S-v2.2	1234 2	1 - COUGH. - LOOSE	99
S-v2.2	1234 2	2 - MIND - RESTLESSNESS	406
S-v2.2	1234 1	3 - COUGH. - DEEP	45
S-v2.2	1234 1	4 - SLEEP - RESTLESS	379
S-v2.2	1234 1	5 - PERSPIRATION. - NIGHT	140
S-v2.2	1234 2	6 - GENERAL - PERSPIRATION, - gives no relief	89
S-v2.2	1234 2	7 - EAR - PAIN - blowing nose,on	16
S-v2.2	1234 2	8 - STOMACH - THIRST - night - waking,on	8
S-v2.2	1234 1	9 - MIND - WEEPING,tearful mood - contradiction,from	4

	1	2	3	4	5	6	7	8	9	10	11	12	13
	stann.	hep.	puls.	calc.	lyc.	con.	ph-ac.	ars.	sep.	stram.	sil.	carb-v.	dig.
	7[a]/12[b]	7/12	6/15	6/13	6/11	6/9	6/7	6/17	6/14	6/12	6/13	6/12	6/10
	[c]11/18	11/17	10/24	10/22	10/17	10/14	10/12	9/26	9/22	9/20	9/19	9/17	9/15
1-	2	1	3	2	1	2	1	3	2	-	2	2	1
2-	2	1	3	3	3	1	2	3	3	3	3	2	2
3-	3	2	-	-	-	-	-	2	1	-	1	2	2
4-	2	2	3	2	3	1	1	3	2	2	3	2	2
5-	1	3	3	2	2	3	1	3	3	1	3	3	1
6-	1	2	2	2	1	1	1	3	3	3	-	1	2
7-	1	1	1	2	1	1	1	-	-	-	1	-	-
8-	-	-	-	-	-	-	-	-	-	2	-	-	-
9-	-	-	-	-	-	-	-	-	-	1	-	-	-

[a] No. of rubrics covered by the remedy.
[b] Total score, based on whether the remedy is plain, italic or bold in each rubric.
[c] Alternative score, taking intensity of the symptom in the case into account.

The child was by nature lean, very thin. She appeared quite weak, as if all the strength had been taken out of her. I did not think of prescribing Stannum until I saw the RADAR analysis and realized it covered the case well. Stannum, of course, is well-known for having an affinity for the respiratory tract and for great weakness. So, I felt optimistic about the prescription. However, as you will see, the remedy did not produce any changes for the better. I probably persisted with Stannum longer than I should have. It was not until two new symptoms appeared on the third day that I saw the correct remedy.

Plan: Stannum metallicum 30c, one dose every two hours.

Follow-Up on Case Number 6

Day 1: No change. Her fever was still 40°C (104°F).

Plan: Continue Stannum.

Day 2: The child was worse. Her fever was sometimes more than 40.5°C (104.9°F); antipyretics were given. Her cough had worsened. Her general state was very weak.

Plan: Continue Stannum.

Day 3: New symptoms developed. She had cold feet with the fever (which continued to be more than 40°C, or 104°F). The child was very difficult to handle; she kicked, hit, tore the house apart, and wept at the slightest provocation.

Plan: Stramonium 30c, one dose every hour until a reaction occurred.

Day 4: Within 12 hours after taking the Stramonium, the picture completely changed. The fever had diminished, and the coughing was less severe. She experienced a gradual and steady improvement from that point on.

Additional Remarks on Case Number 6

The following are other typical symptoms for Stannum:

- Weakness in general, in the chest, and in the respiratory organs; weakness from talking.

- Gradual increasing and decreasing of the pains.

- Short, oppressive breathing, with stitches in the left side of the chest.

- Everything he does causes coughing.

But two new symptoms finally pointed to Stramonium:

- EXTREMITIES: Coldness, foot, fever, during.

- MIND: Destructiveness, kicks, strikes.

In retrospect, it seems that the restlessness in the initial case should lead one to prescribe Stramonium. The VES analysis based on the first set of symptoms had already shown a preference for Stramonium, but this advice was not followed! Stannum seemed the better remedy for a chest problem.

The following is the result of the VES analysis, showing Stramonium as the first possibility:


```
-------------------------------------------HELP IN INTERROGATION-------------------------------------------
    You can question about      1 stram.    2 stann.
    3 ign.      4 apoc.         5 dig.      6 tarent.
    7 hep.      8 coff.         9 ph-ac.    10 mang.
```

Case Number 7

Male, Age 10

Initial Interview: January 4, 1988

He started coughing about a week ago; it had been going up and down, but now his cough is much worse.

His general state is deteriorating rapidly.

He vomited several times from coughing.

The cough increases whenever he lies down, is especially bad around midnight (2), and is better from warm drinks (1).

His fever is 39.8°C (103.7°F).

He looks very ill and "spaced-out."

His movements are slower than usual, and he uses more movements than are necessary. This strange behavior worries his parents a lot.

Analysis of Case Number 7

			No. of remedies in the rubric
S-v2.2	1234	2	1 - STOMACH - VOMITING - coughing,on	76
S-v2.2	1234	2	2 - COUGH. - LYING - agg.	100
S-v2.2	1234	2	3 - COUGH. - NIGHT - midnight	35
S-v2.2	1234	1	4 - COUGH. - WARM, - fluids - amel.	10
S-v2.2	1234	2	5 - MIND - FEAR,apprehension,dread - noise,from	40
S-v2.2	1234	3	6 - HEAD - PAIN,headache in general - noise,from	72
S-v2.2	1234	3	7 - MIND - GROPING as if in the dark	4

	1	2	2	4	5	6	6	8	8	10	11	12	12
	nux-v.	bell.	nit-ac.	phos.	bry.	ars.	sil.	hyos.	lyc.	caust.	cocc.	chin.	nat-c
	$6^a/10^b$	5/8	5/85/8	5/10	5/10	5/10	4/7	5/9	4/7	4/6	4/5	4/5	4/5
	$^c12/19$	11/19	11/19	11/18	10/20	10/19	10/19	10/16	10/16	9/15	9/14	9/12	9/12
1-	2	1	2	1	3	2	2	2	-	-	-	1	1
2-	1	1	1	2	2	2	2	3	2	3	1	-	1
3-	1	1	1	1	1	1	-	-	1	1	1	1	-
4-	3	-	-	-	2	3	3	-	3	-	-	-	-
5-	1	2	1	2	-	-	1	-	2	2	2	1	1
6-	2	3	3	2	2	2	2	1	1	1	2	2	2
7-	-	-	-	-	-	-	-	1	-	-	-	-	-

[a] No. of rubrics covered by the remedy.
[b] Total score, based on whether the remedy is plain, italic or bold in each rubric.
[c] Alternative score, taking intensity of the symptom in the case into account.

This boy lives in another country, and a doctor there had diagnosed the pneumonia. I had successfully treated his chronic asthma problem during the previous two years. His constitutional remedy for the entire two years had been Bryonia. The computer analysis did not strongly suggest any one remedy for the pneumonia, other than perhaps Nux vomica, which was not a clear and obvious choice for me. Because no one remedy stood out for the acute symptoms, I prescribed Bryonia, his constitutional remedy. As you can see, Bryonia generally covers the acute symptoms. This is something I have often done in similar situations, with very good results. And, in this case, the constitutional remedy was able to bring about a rapid and dramatic resolution of the acute illness.

Plan: Bryonia alba 200c, one dose.

Follow-Up on Case Number 7

The remedy was taken the same evening. The next day, all the symptoms were gone. No other dose was needed.

The Constitutional Picture of Bryonia

I would like present a picture of the constitutional Bryonia state. There are some key ideas to keep in mind. One is the idea of security. Security is very important to Bryonia people. They gather things around them and accumulate many possessions. This retention is even represented in their physical appearance, when they retain water during acute illnesses and become puffy. They want to be left alone, not interfered with. The image of the baby in the womb is a useful one for Bryonia. The baby feels comforting pressure all around, and movement is limited. Everything is limited and safe. It is the security of being at home with the mother.

Without this sense of security, Bryonia people can become very anxious. The anxiety can appear in many different areas of life. When they think about health, they are anxious about losing their health. When they think about money, they fear poverty. When they think about the future, they are anxious about losing their current stable situation.

It is interesting to consider the Bryonia alba plant. Above the ground, the plant is beautiful. Below the ground, the plant has a very large bulbous root. The plant stores food and water in this root, always ready for any trouble or disaster that might unexpectedly come along. It is always ready for any change, guarding against any danger or "motion" that might threaten to upset or destroy its world. This plant also has long tendrils, which grow so fast that you can see the growth with the naked eye! These tendrils wrap around everything in a constant effort to consolidate the stability of the plant. In the same way, Bryonia people attach themselves to the surrounding environment, always seeking to anchor their lives and to make sure that nothing will change.

The second important idea in Bryonia is work. Bryonia people are quite focused on work. They are busy working all the time. Work is the way that home and security are maintained. The idea of work appears in many areas — in dreams, delirium, and delusions.

So, we have two big themes: security and work. Many of the physical keynotes can be better understood if these themes are kept in mind. The constipation, for example, is a manifestation of the body keeping all the water, leaving as little to be eliminated as possible and resulting in a hard, dry stool. With a cough, the person holds the chest and tries to keep it still and secure, as if something were about to be lost. With a headache, the person holds the head, stabilizing it against the pain and unsafe situation. And with abdominal pain, Bryonia is better from drawing up the knees. Stretched-out legs produce a vulnerable, open feeling. Drawn-up legs produce a more guarded and protected feeling.

Ananda Zaren, RN

TWO CASES OF PEDIATRIC BEHAVIOR DISORDER

Ananda Zaren, RN, practices in Santa Barbara and Santa Monica, California. She has studied homeopathy since 1977, including extensive studies with George Vithoulkas in the United States and Europe. For the last three years, Ananda has been teaching homeopathy in Holland, England, Belgium, Germany, Norway, and Switzerland. Last year she was invited to work in a German allopathic hospital for four months, where she demonstrated how classical homeopathy could work in a hospital setting. Her base of operations was the obstetrics and gynecology department, where hundreds of clinical videos with follow-ups were made. The success rate was very high. Currently, besides teaching and practicing, Ananda is working on a book.

Case Number 1

Male
Age 6

This is the case of a six-year-old boy who was brought in for homeopathic treatment because he was very aggressive. I am going to be showing a video of my initial interview with the child and his parents. This video was taped at a center in Detmold, Germany, where I have been supervising cases for medical doctors for the last 16 months.

First, I will summarize the doctor's presentation of this case and present the highlights of my initial interview with the child. We will then use the video to analyze the case.

Doctor's Presentation

This boy is extremely aggressive (4). He chokes his parents, his sister, and other children. His sister has to lock herself in her bedroom to hide from his attacks.

He cries very loudly when he does not get his way. He kicks his feet and shrieks for hours at a time. He also curses (1) and destroys things (3). He weeps when he is angry and dislikes any kind of consolation (3).

He thinks he is always right and the best, whatever the situation. He needs a great deal of approval from his parents and constantly asks them, "Is this the right way?" or "Is this all right?"

He is very hyperactive (4); his parents can't understand the power behind him.

When he entered kindergarten, the school asked him to leave because of his aggressiveness. He was violent with the other children and even ripped their clothes off. So far, they will not let him attend classes.

In the night, he always wakes between 1 and 4 a.m., rolls his head from side to side, and moans loudly. He also grinds his teeth in his sleep (2), sleeps on his back, and has nightmares.

The doctors say it must be epilepsy. He was given anticonvulsive drugs, but was taken off of them because they didn't do anything.

His feet perspire. The odor is very offensive. When he takes his shoes off, the smell carries as far as the next room.

He desires sweets (3), ham (3), hot dogs (3), and apple juice (2); he is averse to vegetables (2) and salad (2).

Medical History: Enlarged tonsils; tonsillectomy and adenoidectomy in 1986.

Remedies Given:
- Hyoscyamus 200c in August 1988; no response.
- Tuberculinum 1M in March 1989; no response.

Initial Interview (with Ananda Zaren)

Chief Complaint: aggressive behavior (3). His frustration level is very low. If anything is prohibited, he becomes violent (3).

This aggressive behavior started when he was one year old, after his sister was born. The first symptom that surfaced was a fear of being alone, even for one minute (4). He still has this fear, not only at night but also during the day. He was asked to leave kindergarten because of his aggression and restlessness.

He has angry outbursts (3), curses (1), and hits back strongly (3).

He rolls his head from side to side and moans from 1 to 4 a.m. (3). Has to sleep with a night light (2). He sleeps on his back only (2).

He fears being alone (3) and the dark (2).

He is very rude to everyone, no matter who they are.

Desires cheese (2), mashed apples (2), sausage (2), chicken, (2) fried fish (2), and sweets (2).

Averse to herring (2).

Thirsty. Drinks five cups per day.

Analysis of Case Number 1

[Editors' Note: A video tape was used extensively in this case presentation. We have tried to preserve the style and content of the presentation to help the reader capture its essence without seeing the video.]

[Video run]

> *Zaren: What do you notice?*
>
> *Audience: He looks a bit idiotic. His chin is receding and he looks kind of stupid.*
>
> *Zaren: Anything else?*
>
> *Audience: His eyes are going like a pendulum from side to side.*
>
> *Zaren: Look in the repertory. It's there. And it looks like he is seeing things. At the time, I didn't realize that there was some money on the floor. I want you to see what is happening. This child is checking everything out. Is there anything else that you noticed?*
>
> *Audience: Is the mother holding on to him?*
>
> *Zaren: She puts her hands on his hands.*

[Video run]

Zaren: It is five minutes into the interview, and I heard something peculiar. Did you hear it?

Audience: He is jealous.

Zaren: Yes, but it is peculiar. The parents said that the child cannot be alone for even ten minutes, day or night. I thought to myself, "My God. What is this?" He cannot be alone ever. Now, what else do you notice?

Audience: In addition to moving his eyes from side to side, the tongue comes out.

Zaren: What rubric do you look under for that particular motion?

Audience: It is under MOUTH, motion of the tongue, lapping to and fro.

Zaren: I see four remedies there. The child is very aggressive but cannot be alone. This is the whole focus of the case for me. You are going to find out much more information on the aggressiveness. Also, I want you to watch the father and mother. What are the family dynamics?

[Video run]

Zaren: Is there anything that comes up for you, in terms of remedies and analysis, that fits this picture?

Audience: He is quiet and nice in the chair, especially when the report said that he is hyperactive.

Zaren: The parents said that the hyperactivity came on suddenly, out of nowhere. Are there any remedies that you might think of for this case at the moment?

Audience: Stramonium, because he resembles other hyperactive children, with the violence.

Audience: Tarentula, because of the destructiveness.

Audience: He appears untrustworthy and shifty.

Audience: There is only one remedy for the rubric, lapping of the tongue. Bufo.

Audience: Stramonium, because of the eruption of violence with fear and the fear of being alone.

Audience: Cuprum, because of the lapping of the tongue and the convulsive type of violence.

Audience: Lachesis, because of the lapping of the tongue and the drama.

Zaren: I would like you to decide what you are going to focus on in the case. Are you going to focus on the lapping of the tongue?

Audience: With so many mental symptoms, it might be good to go to GENERALITIES, worse 1 to 4 a.m.

Audience: Stramonium, because there is an alternation of mildness and violence and he is always asking his parents, "Is this the right way?"

Audience: Stramonium, because of his desire for company and because he cannot be alone.

Audience: Bufo, because of the howling and the aggressiveness.

Zaren: Did you see the grimaces? What is your impression?

[Video run]

Audience: I get a feeling that he is experiencing anxiety.

[Video run]

Zaren: Imagine a situation where the family has to change its whole way of functioning because of this boy. He has a lot of power, doesn't he? Very, very smart. Look at how he is sitting so much closer to his mother. There is a little distance with the father. And watch how the child interacts with the father and the mother. It is quite different. The father is very controlling. Soon, the father will completely take over the interview and not let the mother talk. It helps if you can have both parents at your consultations. The child also appears to be moving more when the father is speaking. He seems to be more agitated.

Audience: How are family dynamics helpful in prescribing?

Zaren: You can, perhaps, get the etiology. You need to understand how the patient got to this place in order to understand what is going on at the moment. Was the child abused — emotionally, physically? Is this a fright from the parents, for Hyoscyamus? Is this a disappointed love? Did the father or the mother give no contact?

[Video run]

Zaren: What is the remedy for burrowing the head in the pillow?

Audience: Zincum, because there is so much movement — around the mouth, the rolling of the head, the hyperactivity — and the dullness.

Zaren: We know that he is hyperactive; he doesn't stop moving.

[Video run]

Zaren: Now think about why he moans and tosses his head back and forth between 1 and 4 a.m. It's in the repertory under SLEEP.

Audience: Lycopodium has the rolling of the head from side to side, but it is *day* and *night*.

Zaren: His occurs only in bed.

[Video run]

Zaren: The child resists going to sleep until he is collapsing. It's a fear of being alone. When he causes all this attention by moaning and rolling his head from side to side, his parents come in and take him into their room. So, think about that. It's very important in this case.

Audience: What happened with the Hyoscyamus?

Zaren: The case got worse, then it got better for a short time, and then the whole case relapsed.

[Video run]

Zaren: Again, I hear of his fear of being alone and I think to myself, "My God. He always has to have someone next to him." For me, this is a strange and very peculiar symptom. This is the second time I hear it.

[Video run]

Zaren: When anyone looks from side to side, what is that?

Audience: Suspicion.

Zaren: Yes. Very suspicious.

[Video run]

Zaren: Did you see what just happened? The mother very gently put her hand on the child's legs to let him know that she didn't want him to take the money, and he did it even more. Then the father poked him. The child insists on being watched constantly.

He craves cheese, mashed apples, sausage, hot dogs, fried fish, and sweets. He is averse to herring. He has a thirst for about five glasses a day. So what rubrics would we use here?

Audience: Fears being alone.
Desires company, aggravated alone.
Lacks confidence.
Moans in his sleep.
Laps the tongue.
Destructiveness.
Rolls his head from side to side in sleep.
Perspires. Feet are offensive.
Enlarged tonsils.
Anger with contradiction.
Malicious.
Open mouth.
Shrieks.
Strikes people.
Rudeness.

Zaren: Are there any more candidates for other remedies that we have not included?

Audience: Lycopodium.

Audience: Calcarea phosphorica, because of the enlarged tonsils, moaning, food cravings (smoked meat), violence, and jealousy.

Zaren: The remedy is Gallic acid. I use this particular remedy about two to three times a month. It is not a small remedy.

Clarke has stated in his materia medica:

> Wild delirium at night. Very restless. Jumps out of bed. Sweats profusely. Extremely fearful to be alone. Insists on constantly being watched. Is exceedingly rude and abuses everyone, even his best friends. Jealous of his nurse and curses everyone who speaks to her.

Does it sound like this case? Stramonium didn't seem to fit because there were not as many nightmares and the fear of the dark was hardly there. I know that with Stramonium, the more the unconscious takes over the more the fear of the dark subsides. I had to take that into consideration. But Stramonium has the fear of being alone only at night.

So, Bufo is the differential diagnosis for this case. However, Bufo differs from this case in several ways. Bufo patients get very angry when they are misunderstood. Bufo children and adults bite the flesh on their cuticles and it becomes inflamed. Bufo children act like babies, which is reminiscent of Baryta carbonica or Baryta muriatica. Also, Bufo has a fascination with music. The amelioration is so strong with music, especially classical. Of course, Bufo does have the lapping of the tongue. It also has masturbation or some sexual behavior, which may be present in this case.

My observation in seeing so many of these Gallic acid cases is that they are a cross between Tuberculinum and Stramonium. You will see many symptoms similar to Tuberculinum, such as the tossing of the head from side to side during sleep and the craving for smoked meat. Yet, there is a certain type of violence. The differential factor is this very, very strong fear of being alone. These Gallic acid patients insist on being watched constantly, day and night.

Audience: Is jealousy the main prescribing factor?

Zaren: No, it's not the jealousy. It is the fear of being alone that is the differential. Gallic acid has cursing and jealousy. But the fear of being alone is the big feature in this case.

Audience: Do you ask the adult Gallic acid patient what they are afraid of?

Zaren: Yes. And they do not know. One of my Gallic acid patients has roommates. When they go out he has to have someone come and stay. One roommate was moving out and he would be alone for a couple of weeks. He had to call a housesitting agency to come and stay. This fear is so strong. The violent element of Gallic acid is also strong.

Plan: Gallic acid 200c.

Follow-Up on Case Number 1

First Follow-Up: Two Months After the Remedy

His behavior changed three to four weeks after taking the remedy:

His choking of other people has decreased by 50 to 60 percent.

The rolling of the head and moaning are 50 percent better.

Now he can be alone for small periods of time (1/2 hour).

He is a bit less restless.

His sister does not have to lock herself in a room and hide from his violence.

No night sweats. He still needs a night light.

Desires fried fish (2).

Averse to herring (2).

His rudeness to everyone is much better (80 percent).

He still curses, but it is better.

His therapist has remarked that his concentration and perception have greatly improved.

His frustration level is better.

Plan: Wait.

Fourth Follow-Up: Ten Months After the Remedy

He now can attend classes in school. His behavior at school is very good. His behavior at home is not as good.

He took the remedy in December for four days (D12 potency) and improved greatly.

His tongue is no longer lapping.

Now, he can be alone one hour, which is remarkable according to his mother.

No rolling of the head from side to side and moaning in his sleep.

Night sweats are not as strong. No grinding of the teeth.

His sister no longer has to hide and lock herself up from him.

The choking behavior is better.

The cursing is much improved.

Desires French fries (2), frozen fish (2), and fried sausage (2).

Averse to heavy soup (2) and herring (2).

The rudeness to everyone has improved.

He is now able to fully concentrate.

No hitting and kicking with his feet.

No more need for a night light.

Is still jealous of his sister.

Case Number 2

Male
Age 8

This is the case of an eight-year-old boy who came in for treatment of recurrent sinusitis and hyperactivity. He attends an all-boy day school. He has an 11-year-old sister, and a 20-year-old brother who is no longer living at home. He has a close relationship with his mother but is afraid, at times, of his father. His father has very little patience with him, raises his voice many times, and gets very angry verbally at the boy.

Recurrent sinusitis (2):
- He either has an obstructed or a runny nose (yellow-green discharge) (2). This started one year ago. As a baby, he always had a runny nose with a greenish discharge.
- He had sinus infections eight to nine times in the past year; they were treated with antibiotics.
- Worse from a warm room (2), cold drinks (1), and playing rough (2).
- Better from open air.

Behavior problem:
- His behavior problem started at age two. After he started to crawl and walk, he became very hyperactive (3) and developed an attention disorder (2). He is very aggressive (3) with his sister and with classmates. He constantly gets notes from school; they are deciding what to do. He was put on antidepressants four months ago. They caused many side effects, and he had to be taken off of them.
- He has a problem with concentration (3) and can rarely focus on projects (2).
- He disrupts the whole class (3), spits at and strikes other children (3), curses (1), ignores people when spoken to (2), bites classmates or kicks them (3), initiates all the fights with his classmates and his sister (2), lies (3), is rude to everyone (3), insists on his mother's attention all the time (4), grabs things (3), never says "thank you" or "please" (2), is restless (4), destroys things (3), has no friends

because they are all frightened to be with him, and is jealous (2).
- He fears the dark (2), being alone (3), robbers (2), and ghosts (2).

Desires macaroni and cheese (2), kosher hot dogs (3), pizza (2), and Popsicles (2).

Averse to soup (2), eggs (l), and chicken (2).

Sleep:
- Restless (3).
- Rolls his head from side to side (in second sleep) (2).
- Grinds his teeth (2).
- Has nightmares once a week.
- Has to go to his parents' bedroom to sleep with them every night (3).
- Wakes in the morning refreshed.
- Kicks in his sleep (2).
- Is frightened to stay in his room at night, even with his sister in the same room (3).

Medical History:
- One otitis media at age two.
- Diaper rash and cradle cap as a baby.
- Three colds per year, which always go to the chest.
- Started walking, talking, and teething early.
- Bites his nails frequently (2) and tears off the flesh.

When playing, falls and hurts himself (2). He is constantly in the emergency room (once a week); sprained wrists and arm.

Plan: Gallic acid 200c.

Follow-Up on Case Number 2

First Follow-Up: One Month Later

No episodes of sinusitis in the past month. His nose is now obstructed, but not runny.

His behavior is worse. His parents don't know what to do. His mother feels that homeopathy is not working for her child. His attention span and the hyperactivity are worse.

He is having more difficulty getting to sleep. He comes into his parents' room every night.

His appetite has improved.

To the mother's astonishment, they have not had to go to the emergency room. But she feels this is not due to the homeopathy.

He still bites his nails, but does not bite the cuticle.

Food desires are the same.

Plan: Wait.

Second Follow-Up: Three Months After the Remedy

His sinuses are clear; no yellow-green discharge; no episodes of sinusitis.

His behavior has greatly improved:
- He is much better in school. His parents do not get any notes from the school.
- He is able to focus and concentrate.
- He does not put spiders in jars and try to scare other children.
- When he is reprimanded, he is able to hear it.
- No kicking, spitting, being rude, and striking others.
- Still jealous for attention.

He can now stay alone for 30 minutes.

His nail biting has improved 40 percent.

His sleep is more peaceful. He comes into his parents' room two times a week. No rolling of his head or grinding of his teeth in sleep.

He continues to avoid hurting himself. His mother says that his play is not as rough.

Now, his mother says that she will stay with homeopathy and see what happens.

Plan: Wait.

Third Follow-Up: Seven Months After the Remedy

He continues to do well.

His behavior is 80 percent better.

His attention span is 70 percent better.

His sinus problems are gone.

New symptom: more sloppy in his projects at school and at home.

The mother reports that the child has more self-control and now has one friend. He never gets notes from school.

He has a picky appetite; no new food desires or aversions.

Materia Medica on Gallic Acid

The animal and vegetable kingdom work together to produce Gallic acid. A wasp deposits an egg on a leaf. Something in the egg causes the leaf to secrete a substance that forms a cocoon around the egg to protect it as it grows. Here is a combination of the violence of the wasp and the protection of the leaf.

When the remedy is taken it protects the individual from a deep fear of being alone. As described by Clarke, the main symptoms of Gallic acid are the fear of being alone and the violence in the mental state. The person can be out of control, destructive, and malicious. The destructiveness can be seen by behavior such as biting, kicking, striking, cursing, and destroying things. Gallic acid babies will even kick their feet when they are diapered.

In many ways it can look like a cross between Tuberculinum and Stramonium, but it is neither. You do not feel good about giving either.

Usually the first symptom that will emerge is the fear of being alone. One needs to be aware in studying the materia medica where the focus of the action resides. You will never get this remedy if you do not focus on this strong fear of being alone. There is also a fear of the dark and of ghosts. To differentiate from Stramonium, the fear of being alone is not just at night. It is every minute of the day. In Tuberculinum, the issue is one of dissatisfaction, which is completely different from Gallic acid.

From my Gallic acid cases I have been able to discover that the original cause of this behavior is a sudden shock. The state can come on as the result of a separation from the primary care person. If the child has a predisposition to be Gallic acid, he or she will feel abandoned, for instance, if the mother goes to work. From that time on, the child insists on constantly being watched and never lets the parent out of sight. Adult Gallic acid patients make sure that they live and work with people so that they are never alone.

As with Stramonium, sleep is a very difficult time for Gallic acid. They are restless, kicking and moaning. Children do this to get attention so that they won't have to be alone. It is not enough to have someone in the same room and to have a night light on. They have to be physically next to one of the parents. The children will go to their own bedrooms and fall asleep for a couple of hours. Then they will realize they are alone and will go to the parents' bedroom. They can have bad dreams, but not nightmares like Stramonium where they get up and are frightened, with their eyes wild and wide. They have profuse night sweats like Tuberculinum. The parents will report that these children never have a deep sleep because they are always on guard, watching, so that they are not alone.

In the course of the pathology, we see two characteristic types of behavior. On the one hand, these people are violent, similar to Stramonium. On the other hand, they appear to be quite sweet in front of strangers. In play with other children, they demand to be the center of attention. They are strong leaders. They stir up the other children, and the children become agitated as a defense. They have to win all the time and will cheat at games and at school. They steal toys and then deny it.

The violence of Gallic acid is not directed at themselves but at others, such as peers and family members. They do not bang their heads or injure themselves. The whole family scene has to be changed to accommodate a Gallic acid child; they are very manipulative. There is no privacy for other family members of a Gallic acid patient.

Eight of my cases exhibit compulsive behavior, like Syphilinum, where they touch and smell things. Many times you see the tongue lapping and small bubbles coming out when they talk. They speak in a loud voice, even if they are not angry, and they grimace a lot.

The Gallic acid delirium is described as smashing things, being rude to everyone, cursing. It is a complete mania, with rolling of the head from side to side, biting, kicking, and wild delirium at night. It can look like the anger of Hyoscyamus — sudden and intense. The end result is violent insanity, like Stramonium, except that it does not come on only at night and there is no wild look in their eyes.

The following is a list of rubrics for Gallic acid found in Kent's repertory and in the RADAR synthesized repertory and additions. (RADAR is a computerized repertory program.) Unfortunately, some of the minor remedies, such as Gallic acid, are not represented very well in the repertory. For instance, Gallic acid is not listed under VIOLENCE. Also not listed are a profuse perspiration, a desire for smoked food, and an aversion to herring. I have seen this aversion 27 times.

Kent
1. MIND: Cursing
2. MIND: Jealousy
3. MIND: Jumping, bed, out of
4. MIND: Rudeness (Compare insolent)
5. MIND: Speech, babbling (see MOUTH), strange
6. HEAD: Pain, pain in neck, with
7. NOSE: Roughness inside, posterior nares
8. RECTUM: Hemorrhoids, large
9. RECTUM: Pain, soreness

Synthesis and Additions (RADAR)
1. MIND: Abusive, insulting
2. MIND: Cursing
3. MIND: Delirium
4. MIND: Delirium, bed, escapes, springs up suddenly from
5. MIND: Delirium, wild, night
6. MIND: Desires, full of, watched, to be
7. MIND: Fear, apprehension, dread, solitude of
8. MIND: Irritability
9. MIND: Jealousy
10. MIND: Jumping, bed, out of
11. MIND: Restlessness, night
12. MIND: Rudeness
13. MIND: Speech, strange
14. GENERAL: Convulsions, clonic, epileptiform, absences, petit mal

15. GENERAL: Hemorrhage
16. GENERAL: Weakness, enervation
17. HEAD: Pain, headache in general, pain in neck, with
18. NOSE: Roughness inside, posterior nares
19. RECTUM: Hemorrhoids, large
20. RECTUM: Pain, soreness
21. DREAMS: Amorous
22. DREAMS: Many

NOTES

NOTES

NOTES

NOTES